Color Text of

CONTACT DERMATITIS

Color Text of CONTACT DERMATITIS

Walter G. Larsen, M.D.
Clinical Professor of Dermatology
Oregon Health Sciences University
Portland, Oregon

Robert M. Adams, M.D.
Clinical Professor of Dermatology
Stanford University
Stanford, California

Howard I. Maibach, M.D.
Professor and Vice Chairman
Department of Dermatology
University of California
San Francisco, California

W. B. SAUNDERS COMPANY
Harcourt Brace Jovanovich, Inc.

Philadelphia London Toronto Montreal Sydney Tokyo

W. B. Saunders Company
Harcourt Brace Jovanovich, Inc.

The Curtis Center
Independence Square West
Philadelphia, PA 19106

Library of Congress Cataloging-in-Publication Data

Larsen, Walter G.
Color text of contact dermatitis/Walter G. Larsen, Robert M. Adams, Howard I. Maibach.
p. cm.
Includes index.
ISBN 0-7216-3518-0
1. Contact dermatitis—Atlases. I. Adams, Robert M., II. Maibach, Howard I. III. Title.
[DNLM: 1. Dermatitis, Contact—atlases. WR 17 L334c]
RC593.C6L37 1992
616.5'1'0222—dc20
DNLM/DLC 91-28791

Editor: W. B. Saunders Staff
Designer: Maureen Sweeney
Production Manager: Peter Faber
Manuscript Editors: Tina K. Rebane and Karen Okie
Illustration Coordinator: Brett MacNaughton
Indexer: Roger Wall
Cover Designer: Michelle Maloney

Color Text of Contact Dermatitis ISBN 0-7216-3518-0

Printed in MEXICO.

Last digit is the print number: 9 8 7 6 5 4 3 2 1

Contributors

Donald V. Belsito, M.D.
Associate Professor of Dermatology, New York University Medical Center, New York, New York
The Mechanism of Allergic Contact Dermatitis

Joseph F. Fowler, Jr., M.D.
Assistant Professor of Dermatology, University of Louisville School of Medicine, Louisville, Kentucky
How to Patch Test

Clifton R. White, Jr., M.D.
Professor of Dermatology and Pathology, Oregon Health Sciences University, Portland, Oregon
Dermatopathology of Contact Dermatitis

Foreword

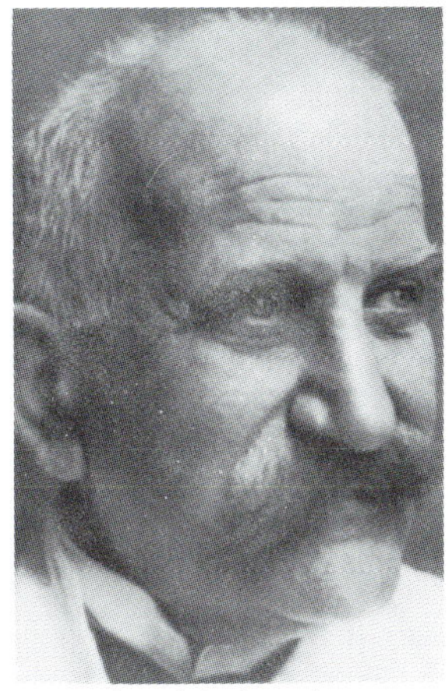

Josef Jadassohn
(1863–1936)

A History of Contact Dermatitis: Josef Jadassohn (1863–1936)

It was a chance observation that resulted in the discovery of a new, important diagnostic tool, the patch test. In 1896, Professor Josef Jadassohn, then Chief of Dermatology at the Allerheiligen Hospital in Breslau, Germany, was treating a young man for pediculosis pubis with the commonly used mercury-containing "blue ointment." After approximately 24 hours, the patient developed a severe eczematous eruption at the site of application. Jadassohn reasoned that the entire skin was sensitized and that application of the ointment to a small area of uninvolved skin would reproduce the eruption. Jadassohn termed his test "junctionelle Hautprüfung," or junctional skin test. This became the basis for the so-called patch test.

Thus, Jadassohn was the first to conclude that in certain eczematous and erythematous dermatoses, the eruption depended on specific sensitization of the skin, and that proof could be established by the simple application of the suspected substance, in nonirritating concentration, to a small area of unaffected, grossly normal skin.

This important contribution to medicine was only one of many for this remarkable man. Jadassohn possessed an astounding knowledge of almost every aspect of medicine and biology, and he combined this knowledge with an extraordinary breadth of vision. Among his most enduring subjects of investigation, besides the genesis of eczema, were the morphology and immunology of tuberculosis of the skin; the histology and genesis of congenital anomalies; extensive research on venereal diseases, fungal diseases, leprosy, and immunology; drug eruptions; the use of laboratory aids such as complement fixation tests; and cultural methods of diagnosis. He was an indefatigable worker and shared his vast knowledge as the author of the great 41-volume *Handbuch der Haut- und Geschlechtskrankheiten* and as the editor of the *Archiv für Dermatologie und Syphilis* and the *Zentralblatt für Haut- und Geschlechtskrankheiten*.

Jadassohn is one of the great scientists and clinicians in the history of dermatology. As the founder of the patch test, we salute him and dedicate this book to his memory.

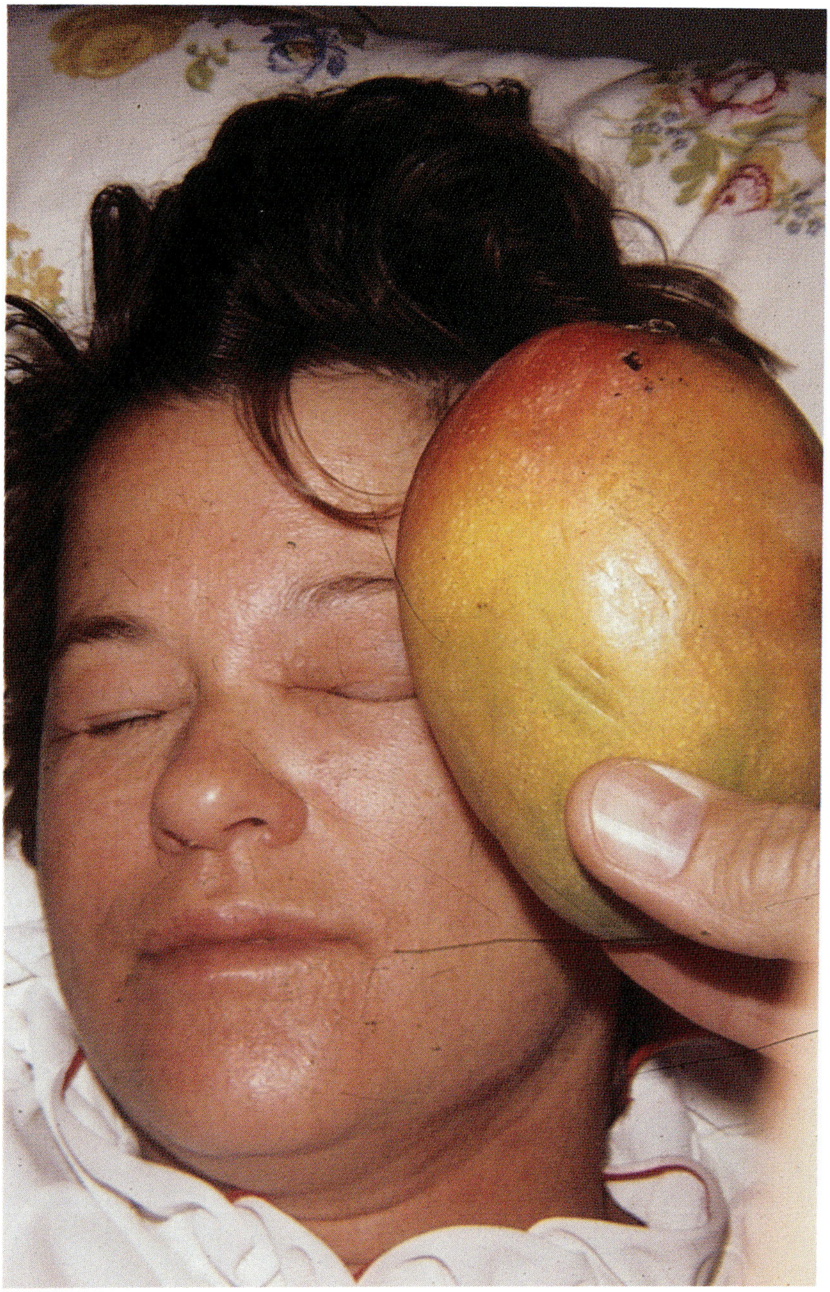

Preface

The authors of this book hope that by its publication physicians will be encouraged and perhaps enticed to enter the exciting and challenging world of contact dermatitis. The two standard textbooks on contact dermatitis* today are excellent sources of information, but neither contains a single photograph! In preparation of *Color Text of Contact Dermatitis*, we have juxtaposed a representative photograph or two with the most important information in capsule form and have avoided lengthy discourses on diagnosis and treatment. The conditions discussed range from the common to the unusual. An important section concerns those diseases that closely mimic contact dermatitis. The references included are those we considered to be the most representative and current.

A photograph brings to reality a concept and fixes it in the consciousness. Centuries ago, the Chinese realized this, as inscribed in their well-known proverb: "A picture is worth a thousand words." We believe this is still true today and are presenting this book with this aphorism as our guide.

WALTER G. LARSEN, M.D.
ROBERT M. ADAMS, M.D.
HOWARD I. MAIBACH, M.D.

---

* Fisher AA: Contact Dermatitis, 3rd ed. Philadelphia, Lea & Febiger, 1987.
Cronin E: Contact Dermatitis. Edinburgh, Churchill Livingstone, 1980.

Contents

Chapter 1

The Mechanism of Allergic Contact Dermatitis

DONALD V. BELSITO, MD

As classified by Coombs and Gell,[1] allergic contact dermatitis (ACD) represents a Type IV cell-mediated reaction. At the time that this classification system was proposed, the skin was thought to be an inert barrier to the external environment passively injured by immunologic responses to contact allergens. Much work during the past decade has shown that the skin is an active participant in the allergic response. Indeed, most environmental contact allergens are low molecular weight molecules (haptens) that, before they can sensitize, must be processed and covalently linked to proteins to form a complete antigen.[2] This "processing" of the low molecular weight allergen is performed by the Langerhans cells (LCs), the antigen-presenting cells (APCs) of the skin.

LCs are bone marrow–derived dendritic cells situated within the suprabasilar layer of the epidermis; they constitutively express Class II (HLA-DR) antigens on their surface.[3] Because of their limited capability for phagocytosis, antigen processing by the LCs most likely involves endocytosis, degradation of the antigen, and recycling of antigenic fragments bound to HLA-DR onto their surface.[4] It is the linkage of the hapten to HLA-DR molecules that makes it a complete antigen.

In order for an allergic response to occur, LCs not only must process the antigen, but must then present it to CD4$^+$ T cells (T helper cells) with receptors specific for HLA-DR antigen and the contact allergen (Fig. 1–1). The antigen-specific receptor on T cells consists of CD3, a surface-transducing protein found on all T cells, linked to Ti, a protein whose variable regions act as the specific antigen-binding site.[5] In addition to the CD3-Ti complex, CD4 antigen on helper T cells acts as an additional recognition site for HLA-DR on APCs. Thus, ACD can occur only if the APC expresses HLA-DR molecules on its surface.[6] Whether this LC-T cell interaction occurs in the skin (peripheral presentation) or in the paracortical (thymus-dependent) areas of the draining lymph nodes (central presentation) is a matter of continued controversy (reviewed in reference 7).

The role that epidermal cells play in ACD is not limited to processing and presentation of the antigen. As LCs interact with CD3-Ti$^+$,CD4$^+$ lymphocytes, interleukin-1 (IL-1) is synthesized and released by LCs[8] and, perhaps, by keratinocytes.[9] In ACD, the primary function of IL-1 is to activate T cells to

Dr. Belsito is the recipient of a Clinical Investigator Award from the NIAMS No. AR-01439.

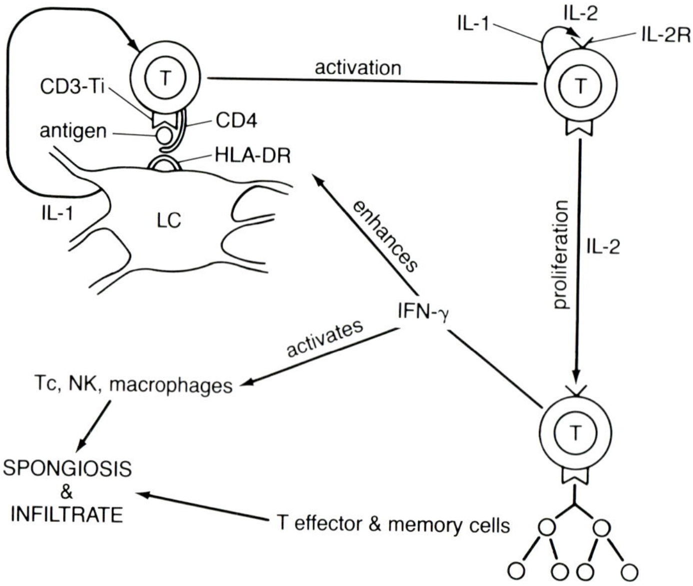

Figure 1–1 An overview of the mechanism of allergic contact dermatitis. See text for details. CD3-Ti—antigen recognition site; CD4—a recognition site for HLA-DR; HLA-DR—Class II antigen; IFN-γ—gamma-interferon; IL—interleukin; IL-2R—IL-2 receptor; LC—Langerhans cells; NK—natural killer cells; T—T cells; Tc—cytotoxic T cells. (From Belsito D: The pathophysiology of allergic contact hypersensitivity. Clin Rev Allergy 7: 347, 1989.)

produce and secrete interleukin-2 (IL-2). Together with IL-1, IL-2 induces its own receptor (IL-2R) on T cells. Although IL-2 is a product of specifically sensitized $CD4^+$ T cells, it acts nonspecifically to stimulate $CD4^+$ and $CD8^+$ (cytotoxic and suppressor) T cells, with and without specific antigen receptors, to express IL-2R, to proliferate in response to IL-2, and to secrete gamma-interferon (IFN-γ).[10] Thus, the final response to a contact allergen is nonspecific, although the $CD4^+$,$CD3\text{-}Ti^+$ T cells do localize ACD to the site of challenge via their site-specific production of IL-2 and IFN-γ. It is IFN-γ, in conjunction with IL-2, that activates cytotoxic T cells, natural killer (NK) cells, and macrophages.[11] These cells, along with their soluble mediators, eventuate in epidermal edema (spongiosis) and dermal infiltrate, which, although not diagnostic, are characteristic of ACD (Fig. 1–2).

Although the current dogma is that IL-1, IL-2, and IFN-γ are the primary mediators of ACD, other epidermal cytokines will undoubtedly be shown to play a prominent role in the reaction. IFN-γ induces the production of tumor necrosis factor (TNF) by monocytes[12] and, most likely, by LCs.[13] TNF is a

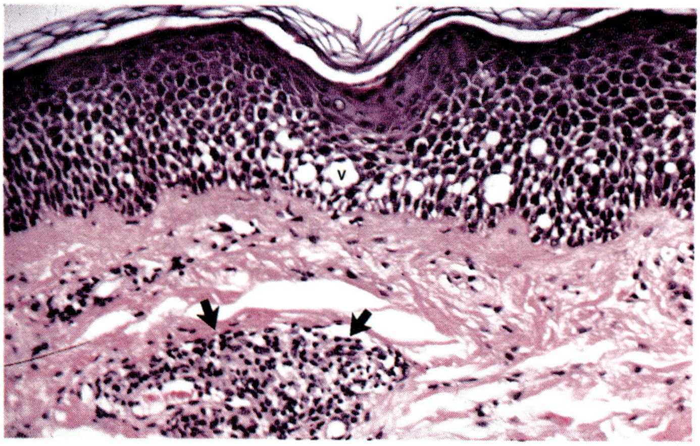

Figure 1–2 Histopathology of allergic contact dermatitis. A biopsy of the eruption shows epidermal intercellular edema and microvesiculation (*v*), which are characteristic of an allergic response as well as of other eczematous dermatitides. The superficial perivascular infiltrate (*arrows*) consists of lymphocytes, macrophages, and occasionally eosinophils.

cytokine that can produce necrosis of selected tumor lines—hence its name. TNF is also known to enhance antigen-induced T cell proliferation.[14] Furthermore, both TNF and IL-1 induce interleukin-6 (IL-6),[15] a product of a variety of cell types including keratinocytes.[16] IL-6 is known to upregulate Class II antigen on LCs[17] and to function as a second signal for IL-2 production by mature T cells.[18] In addition to IL-6, keratinocytes make a variety of other immunologically important molecules including interleukin-8 (IL-8), a potent chemoattractant for neutrophils and lymphocytes.[19] Thus, it is likely that future studies will show that other epidermal cytokines (such as TNF, IL-6, IL-8, and others) contribute to the final pathologic changes seen in ACD.

Recently, several reports have shown that mast cells are also activated during ACD, most likely by a T cell–derived antigen-binding factor.[20] In mice, this factor causes mast cells to release serotonin within 2 hours after antigenic challenge. Other investigators have noted a triphasic cutaneous allergic response in mice following antigenic challenge. The allergic reaction peaked at 1.5, 8, and 24 hours and was associated with elevated serum histamine levels at 1 to 4, 12, and 48 hours. If, as suggested,[20,21] vasoactive amines are important regulators of ACD via their induction of endothelial gaps that permit the ingress or egress of effector cells, the first two peaks at 1 to 4 and 12 hours would be of greatest relevance since they more closely correspond to the appearance of the cellular infiltrate, which begins as early as 2 to 4 hours and peaks at 24 hours following challenge with an offending allergen.[21] The presence of a third peak of histamine at 48 hours,[21] a time of decreased responsiveness, suggests that histamine, which is known to exert a stimulatory effect on suppressor T lymphocytes,[22] may be involved in downregulating the reaction in the later stages. Basophils may play a similar role in downregulating sensitivity since, in humans, 5 to 15% of the infiltrating cells in waning allergic reactions are basophils.[23] The involvement of mast cells and basophils in ACD may explain the concurrence of urticaria and eczema, as noted in certain allergic responses such as "protein contact dermatitis."[24]

Once an allergic reaction ensues, a variety of factors come into play to terminate the reaction. Chief among these are desquamation of antigen-laden skin and cellular or enzymatic degradation of antigen with destruction of the APCs. In addition, other regulatory mechanisms contribute to the resolution of the allergic response. As previously mentioned, mast cell- and basophil-derived histamine can activate suppressor T cells. Furthermore, in response to stimulation by IFN-γ, macrophages produce prostaglandins (PGs), especially of the E series.[25] Both PGE_1 and PGE_2 inhibit production of IL-2 and expression of the IL-2R.[26] Thus, soluble mediators such as histamine or PG, which are responsible for eliciting the reaction, also play an active role in dampening the response.

Despite the gains in our understanding of the mechanism of ACD during the past decade, much work remains to be done. For the years 1984 to 1985, the most frequent contact allergens in the United States included nickel, paraphenylenediamine, Quaternium-15, neomycin, thimerosal, formaldehyde, cinnamic aldehyde, ethylenediamine, potassium dichromate, and thiurams.[27] However, the dynamics of percutaneous absorption of these chemicals and the nature of the antigenic moiety within them remain unknown. Such knowledge would be useful in the production of effective barrier creams and in the development of more reliable *in vivo* and *in vitro* diagnostic tests for ACD. Delineation of the complex interactions between LCs and T cells, as well as between the various soluble mediators of cellular immunity, should further our understanding of those factors that enhance or diminish ACD. With the advent of such information, new therapies, including successful hyposensitization, should be available to physicians of the twenty-first century.

References

1. Coombs RRA, Gell PGH: Classification of allergic reactions responsible for clinical hypersensitivity and disease. In Gell PGH, Coombs RRA, Lachman LB (eds): Clinical Aspects of Immunology, 3rd ed. Oxford, Blackwell Scientific Publications, 1975, p 761.
2. Landsteiner K, Chase MW: Studies on the sensitization of animals with simple chemical compounds: IX. Skin sensitization induced by injection of conjugates. J Exp Med 73:431, 1941.
3. Rowden G, et al: Ia antigen expression on human epidermal Langerhans cells. Nature (Lond) 268:247, 1977.
4. Hanau D, et al: Human epidermal Langerhans cells cointernalize by receptor-mediated endocytosis "nonclassical" major histocompatibility complex class I molecules (T6 antigens) and class II molecules (HLA-DR antigens). Proc Natl Acad Sci USA 84:2901, 1987.
5. Reinherz EL, et al: The delineation of antigen receptors on human T lymphocytes. Immunol Today 4:5, 1983.
6. Schwartz RH: T lymphocyte recognition of antigen in association with gene products of the major histocompatibility complex. Annu Rev Immunol 3:237, 1985.
7. Belsito DV: The pathophysiology of allergic contact hypersensitivity. Clin Rev Allergy 7:347, 1989.
8. Sauder DN, et al: Langerhans cell production of interleukin-1. J Invest Dermatol 82:605, 1984.
9. Luger TA, et al: Murine epidermal cell-derived thymocyte-activating factor resembles murine interleukin 1. J Immunol 128:2147, 1982.
10. Chang TW, et al: Cellular origin and interactions involved in gamma-interferon production induced by OKT3 monoclonal antibody. J Immunol 128:585, 1982.
11. Vilcek J, et al: Interferon-gamma: A lymphokine for all seasons. Lymphokines 11:1, 1985.
12. Beutler B, et al: Effect of gamma-interferon on cachectin expression by mononuclear phagocytes. Reversal of the lps^d (endotoxin resistance) phenotype. J Exp Med 164:1791, 1986.
13. Larrick JW, et al: Activated Langerhans cells release tumor necrosis factor. J Leukocyte Biol 45:429, 1989.
14. Yokota S, et al: Enhancement of antigen- and mitogen-induced human T lymphocyte proliferation by tumor necrosis factor-alpha. J Immunol 140:531, 1988.
15. Ray A, et al: Activation of the human "beta$_2$-interferon/hepatocyte stimulating factor/interleukin 6" promoter by cytokines, viruses, and second messenger agonists. Proc Natl Acad Sci USA 85:6701, 1988.
16. Kirnbauer R, et al: IFN-beta 2, B cell differentiation factor 2, or hybridoma growth factor (IL-6) is expressed and released by human epidermoid cells and epidermoid carcinoma cell lines. J Immunol 142:1922, 1989.
17. Belsito DV, et al: Enhancement by various cytokines and beta mercaptoethanol of Ia antigen expression on Langerhans cells in skin from normal aged and young mice: Effect of cyclosporine A. J Immunol 143:1530, 1989.
18. Garman RD, et al: B-cell stimulatory factor 2 (beta$_2$ interferon) functions as a second signal for interleukin 2 production by mature murine T cells. Proc Natl Acad Sci USA 84:7629, 1987.
19. Larsen CG, et al: The neutrophil activating protein (NAP-1) is also chemotactic for lymphocytes. Science 243:1464, 1989.
20. Askenase PW, et al: T cells produce an antigen-binding factor with *in vivo* activity analogous to IgE antibody. J Exp Med 157:862, 1982.
21. Kerdel FA, et al: Mast cell participation during the elicitation of murine allergic contact hypersensitivity. J Invest Dermatol 88:686, 1987.
22. Sahasrabudhe DK, et al: Inhibition of suppressor T lymphocytes (Ts) by cimetidine. J Immunol 138:2760, 1987.
23. Dvorak HF, et al: Morphology of delayed-type hypersensitivity reactions in man. J Invest Dermatol 67:391, 1976.
24. Hjorth N, Roed-Petersen J: Occupational protein contact dermatitis in food handlers. Contact Dermatitis 2:28, 1976.
25. Gemsa D: Stimulation of prostaglandin E release from macrophages and possible role in the immune response. In Pick E (ed): Lymphokines. New York, Academic Press, 1981, p 335.
26. Walker C, et al: Lymphokine regulation of activated (G1) lymphocytes. Prostaglandin E2-induced inhibition of interleukin 2 production. J Immunol 130:1770, 1983.
27. Storrs FJ, et al: Prevalence and relevance of allergic reactions in patients patch tested in North America—1984 to 1985. J Am Acad Dermatol 20:1038, 1989.

Chapter 2

Dermatopathology of Contact Dermatitis

CLIFTON R. WHITE, JR., MD

Contact dermatitis has a variety of clinical expressions, each with characteristic histologic features.[1-5] Allergic contact dermatitis (ACD) and irritant contact dermatitis (ICD) (nonimmune-mediated) are common. Less frequently encountered types include photoallergic and phototoxic contact dermatitis, contact urticaria, and rarely "contact dermatitis" provoked by systemic agents.[6]

Spongiosis, or intercellular edema between epidermal spinous cells, is the histologic hallmark of ACD. In early ACD, the amount of spongiosis may be minimal to moderate, within a normal-thickness epidermis, accompanied by a superficial perivascular infiltrate of lymphocytes, histiocytes, and usually eosinophils. As epidermal edema accumulates, keratinocytes may become separated, forming microscopic or clinically visible vesicles (and occasionally bullae), with pallor of the papillary dermis. Scale crust (plasma, parakeratosis, and inflammatory cells) within the stratum corneum, erosions, and ulcerations may also be present (Fig. 2–1).

As clinical lesions persist, the histologic features of ACD evolve (subacute), with the hallmark spongiosis typically present within a thickened epidermis, accompanied by coarse collagen-replacing edema within the papillary dermis. Long-standing lesions (chronic) may eventually show only residua of spongiosis (scale crust) in the stratum corneum, with irregular epidermal hyperplasia overlying a thickened, fibrotic papillary dermis.

Irritant contact dermatitis (ICD) progresses through clinical and histologic stages similar to those in ACD, often accompanied by intracellular edema (ballooning) as well as spongiosis, at times leading to reticular change ("degeneration"), in addition to epidermal necrosis. The inflammatory infiltrate in ICD may contain neutrophils as well as lymphocytes, histiocytes, and eosinophils (Fig. 2–2). Despite these subtle histologic differences, ACD cannot reliably be distinguished from ICD microscopically.

The histopathologic features seen in biopsies of patch test reactions often mimic those of the original dermatitis.

Contact dermatitis elicited by light exposure (photoallergic and phototoxic contact dermatitis) has histologic features similar to those of ACD and ICD, often with dyskeratotic keratinocytes ("sunburn cells") and an inflammatory infiltrate extending to the deep reticular dermis.

Contact urticaria lacks the epidermal changes seen in allergic and irritant contact dermatitis and their photorelated counterparts (photoallergic and phototoxic dermatitis). Rather, contact urticaria is characterized histologically by a superficial or superficial and deep perivascular and interstitial mixed cellular infiltrate of lymphocytes, mast cells, eosinophils, and neutrophils—the last two often scattered between collagen bundles.

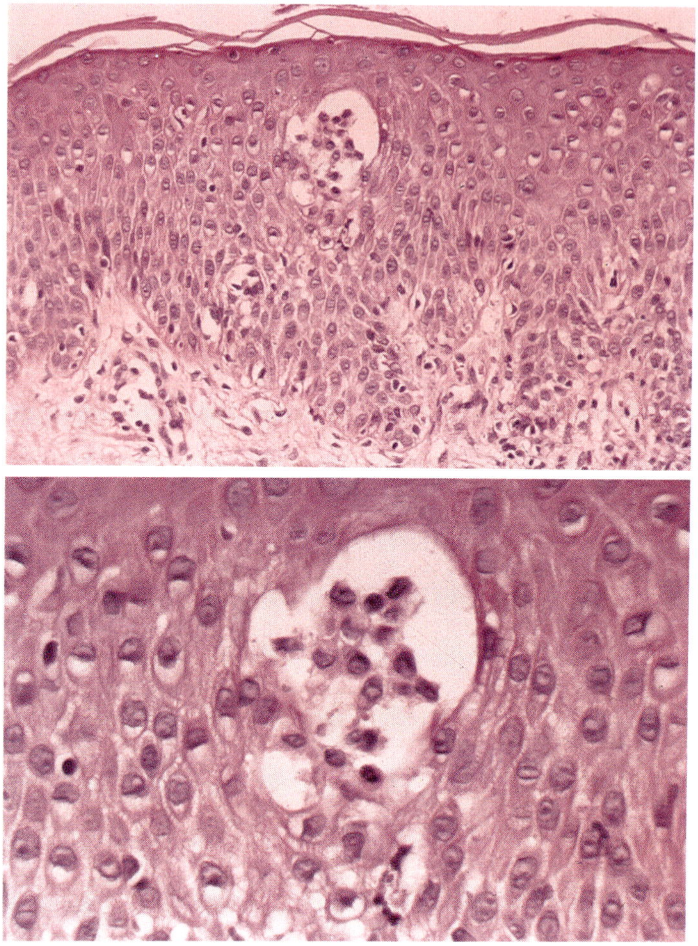

A

B

Figure 2–1 (*A*) Allergic contact dermatitis (ACD), subacute. Note the spongiotic microvesicle within a slightly hyperplastic epidermis, some adjacent intercellular edema, papillary dermal fibrosis, and a superficial perivascular and interstitial mixed inflammatory infiltrate consisting predominantly of lymphocytes and eosinophils. Similar changes are often seen in irritant contact dermatitis, frequently with neutrophils as a major component of the infiltrate. (*B*) High power magnification of the spongiotic microvesicle containing lymphocytes. Note some separation of surrounding keratinocytes (spongiosis), making intercellular bridges (desmosomes) more apparent.

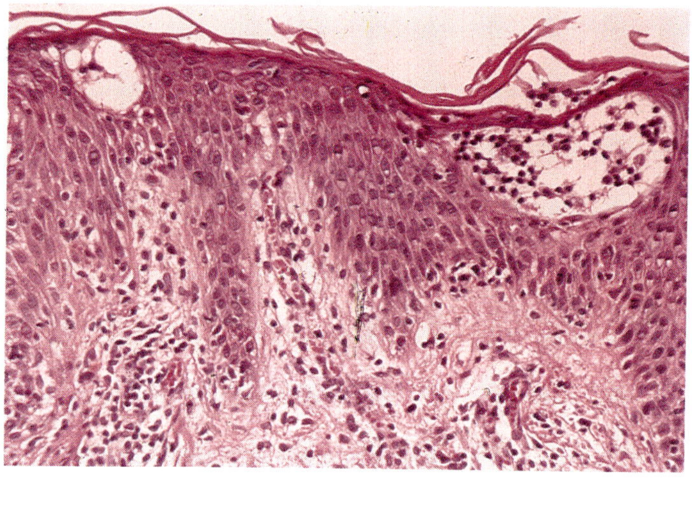

Figure 2–2 Irritant contact dermatitis (ICD). Note the similarity to changes seen in Figure 2–1, including multiple spongiotic microvesicles associated with lymphocytes. Ballooning, or intracellular edema, is also present, along with occasional necrotic keratinocytes and a superficial infiltrate including neutrophils and eosinophils. Consistent histologic distinction between ACD and ICD is usually not possible.

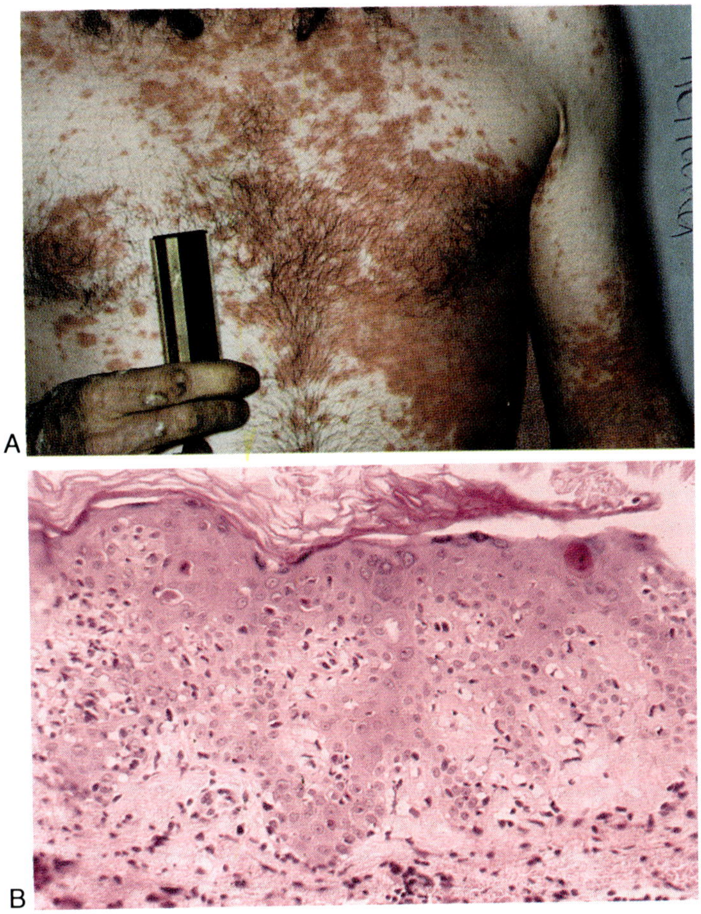

Figure 2–3 (*A*) Clinical photograph of a patient (holding a piece of rosewood) who, while doing cabinetry work, developed contact erythema multiforme from shavings of rosewood. (*B*) Biopsy specimen from the same patient showing erythema multiforme-like changes, including vacuolar alteration of the basal layer with numerous necrotic keratinocytes and a superficial perivascular lymphocytic infiltrate. The patient also had a positive patch test for rosewood; a biopsy specimen from the reaction site showed histologic features similar to those of erythema multiforme. No spongiosis was present in either biopsy.

The histologic changes of "systemic" contact dermatitis are, most often, similar to those described for ACD, with spongiosis the predominant feature.[6] Other quite rare clinical presentations of systemic contact dermatitis include erythema multiforme[7,8] (Fig. 2–3), vasculitis, bullae, granulomas, stomatitis, and erythroderma, each with corresponding histology.

References

1. Lever WF, Schaumberg-Lever G: Histopathology of the Skin, 7th ed. Philadelphia, JB Lippincott, 1989.
2. Ackerman AB: Histologic Diagnosis of Inflammatory Skin Diseases. Philadelphia, Lea & Febiger, 1978.
3. Hjorth N, Fregert S: Contact dermatitis. In Rook A, Wilkinson DS, Ebbling FJG (eds): Textbook of Dermatology, 3rd ed. Oxford, Blackwell Scientific Publications, 1979.
4. Ackerman AB: Histologic findings in different types of contact dermatitis. In Fisher A: Contact Dermatitis, 3rd ed. Philadelphia, Lea & Febiger, 1986.
5. Taylor RM: Histopathology of contact dermatitis. Clin Dermatol 4:18–22, 1986.
6. White CR, Jr: Histopathology of exogenous and systemic contact eczema. Semin Dermatol 9:1–3, 1990.
7. Irvine C, Reynolds A, Finlay AY: Erythema multiforme-like reaction to "rosewood." Contact Dermatitis 14:224–225, 1988.
8. Holst R, Kirby J, Magnusson B: Sensitization to tropical woods giving erythema multiforme-like eruptions. Contact Dermatitis 2:295–296, 1976.

Chapter 3

How to Patch Test

JOSEPH F. FOWLER, JR., MD

A key to successful patch testing, in addition to the proper selection of patients and allergens, is correct patch-testing technique. The steps involved include preparation, placement, and later removal of the patches; reading the tests; and interpretation of the results. The Finn Chambers on Scanpor tape is the current standard patch set most commonly used worldwide (Figs. 3–1 and 3–2). The True-Test kit offers a new patch, and it is supplied with allergens already in place.

PREPARATION OF THE PATCH

Preparing the patches is illustrated in Figures 3–3 through 3–5. Allergens in petrolatum are applied directly to the aluminum disc. An amount sufficient to fill the chamber slightly more than one-half full should be used. For allergens in water or other liquids, a tiny spot of petrolatum is placed on the chamber, followed by a filter paper disc. Then one drop of the allergen solution is applied to the disc. For ease in transporting the patch from the preparation area to the patient, the backing paper may be carefully placed back on the patch and removed at the time of application.

The True-Test kit consists of a series of patches with allergens suspended in a gel vehicle already affixed to the tape. No further preparation is necessary (Fig. 3–6).

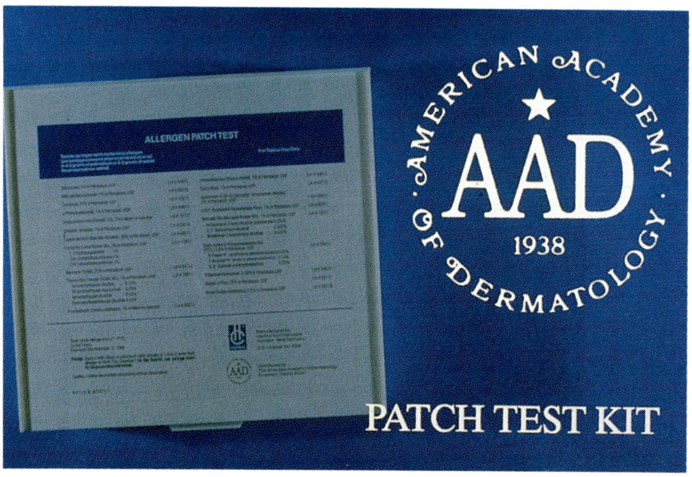

Figure 3–1 Current standard tray of 20 screening substances.

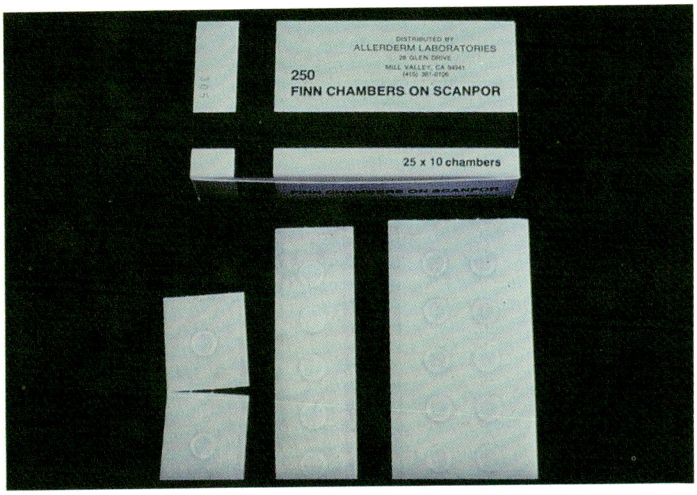

Figure 3–2 Finn Chambers on Scanpor tape are supplied singly and in strips of five or ten discs.

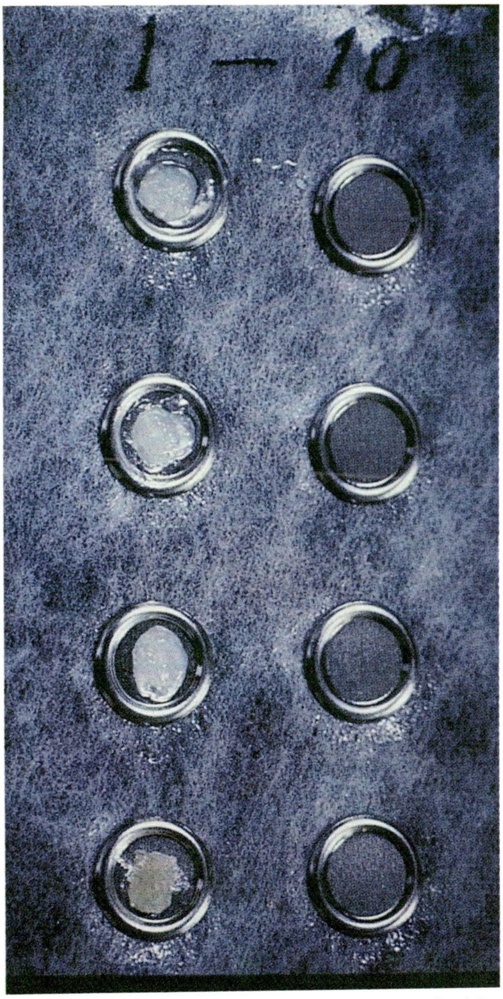

Figure 3–3 Allergens in petrolatum are applied to the discs.

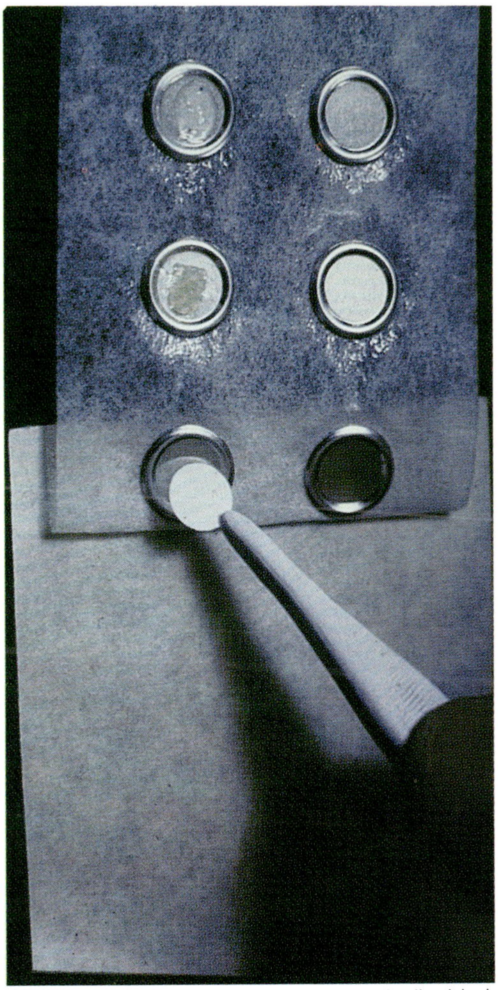

Figure 3–4 Filter paper discs are used for liquid allergens.

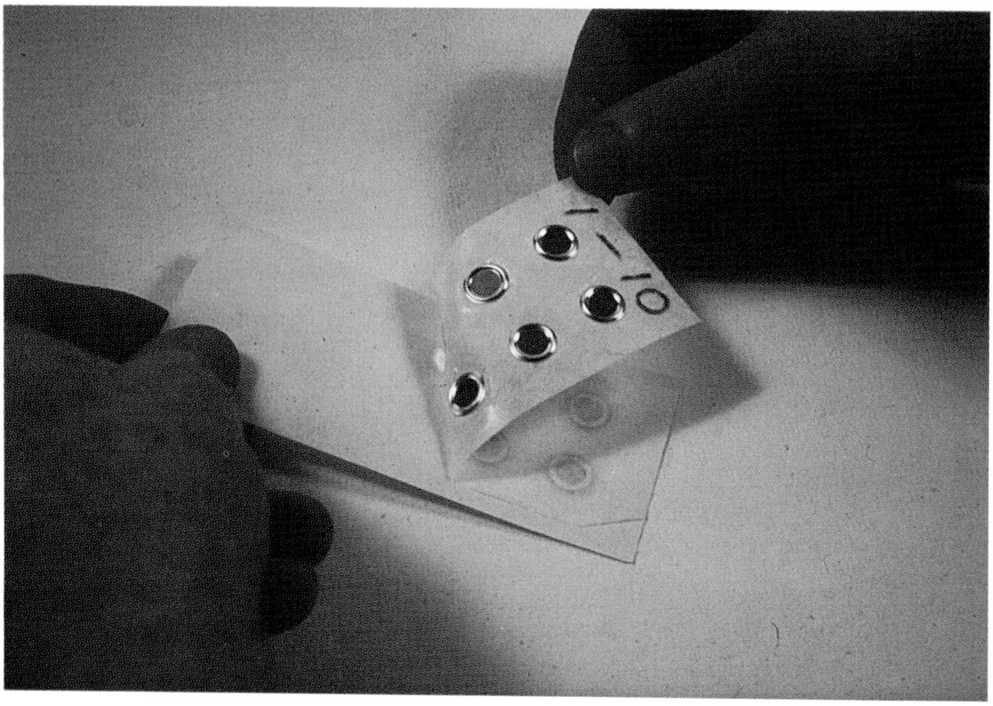

Figure 3–5 The backing paper is reapplied to the patches for transportation.

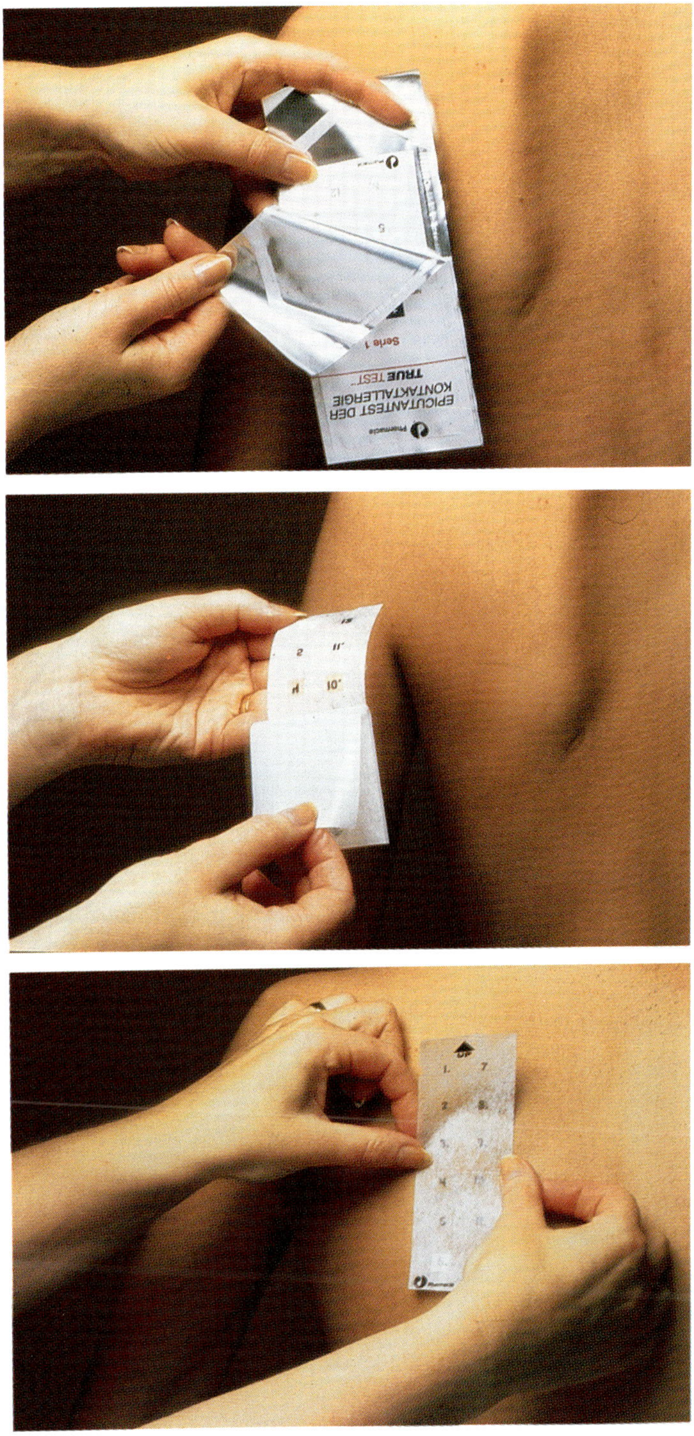

A

B

C

Figure 3–6 (*A, B, C*) The True-Test is a factory-prepared allergen patch that requires no preparation. The patch is applied straight from the package.

PLACEMENT OF THE PATCH TESTS

Proper application of the patches to the skin is essential for accurate patch test interpretation. Proper technique is shown in Figure 3-7.

Tests should be applied on an area of the upper back free of dermatitis and hair; if necessary, shaving with an electric razor may be done. Shaving cream or soap should not be used. Placement of patches over a pigmented nevus or similar lesion should be avoided because of possible irritation of the lesion and difficulty in reading the test. Vertical strip positioning results in better adherence to the skin. Careful strip placement prevents accidental intermixing of substances. After the strips are in place, the tester should run a hand over them to disperse the substances and ensure adherence. Do not over-tape.

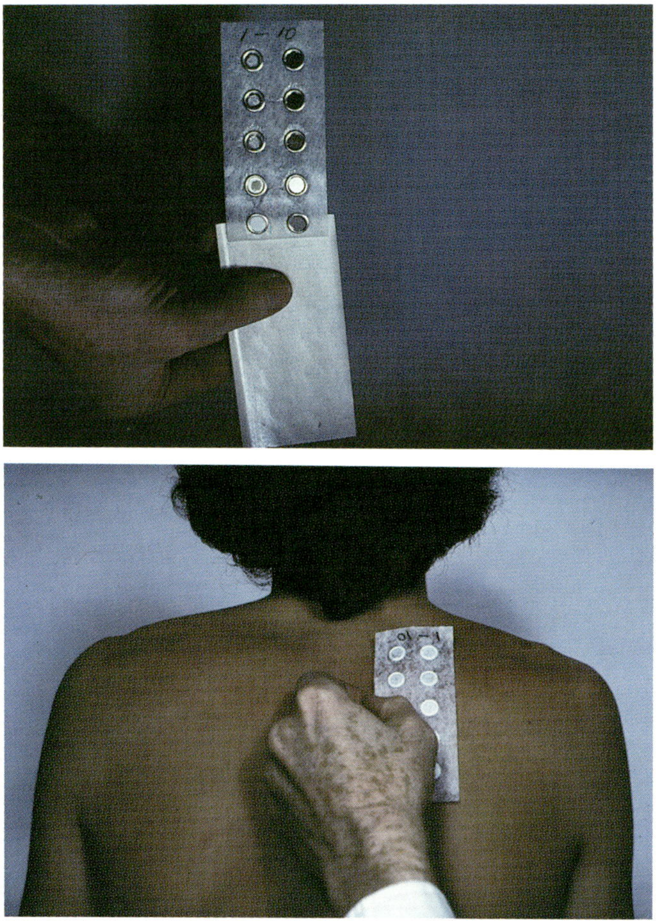

A

B

Figure 3-7 (*A* to *E*) Finn Chambers. After the backing paper is removed, the patches are applied to the patient's back.

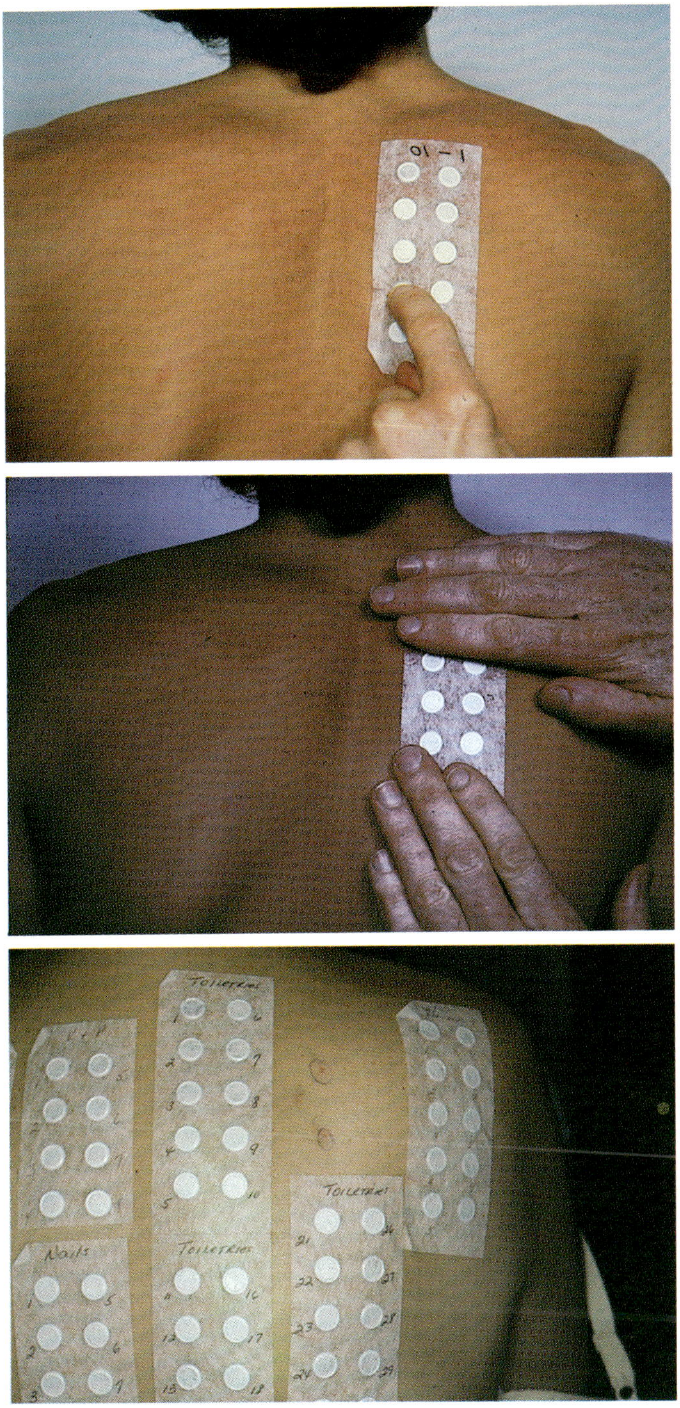

C

D

E

Figure 3–7 *Continued*

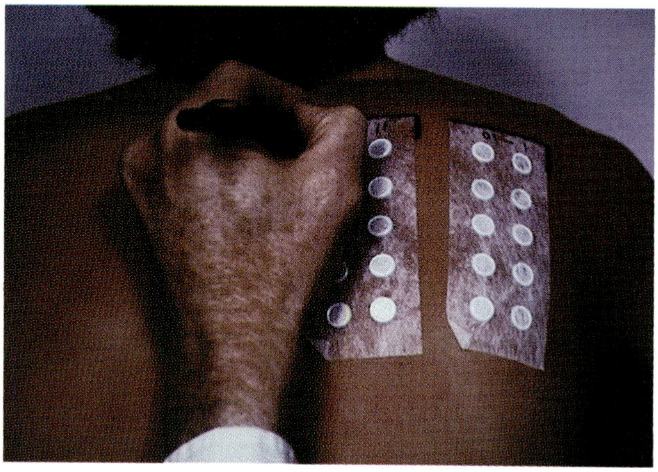

Figure 3–8 Patches in place. Note that one corner is turned under for easy removal. Avoid placing patches over acne papules, nevi, or other lesions that may confuse the reading.

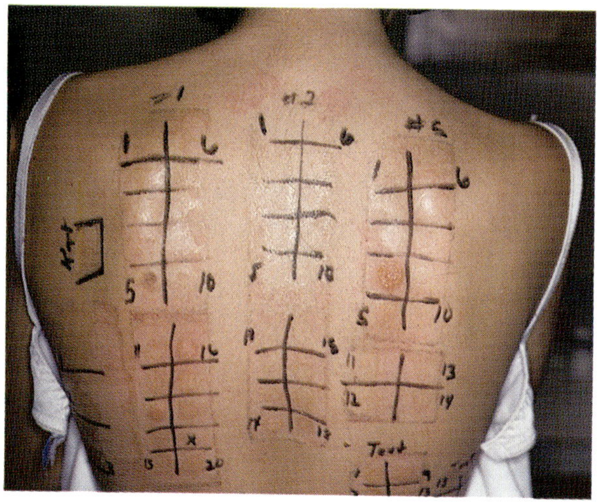

Figure 3–9 Patches are off and the patient's back is marked. Dark ink facilitates immediate reading, whereas fluorescent ink is helpful for a later reading.

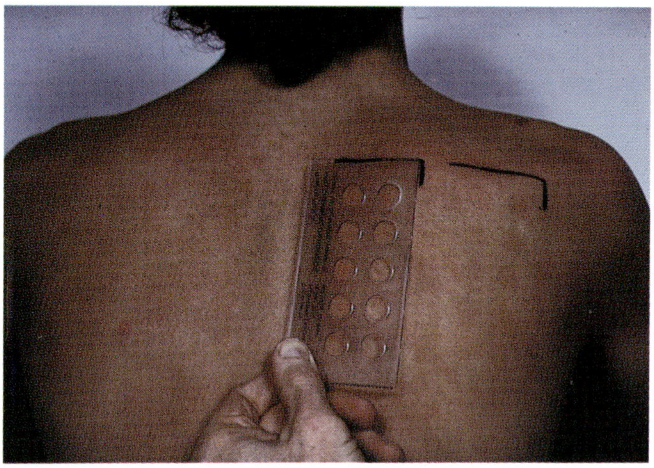

Figure 3–10 Use of a template in identifying patches.

Table 3–1. NACDG PATCH TEST GRADING SYSTEM

0 or –	No reaction
?	Macular erythema only
1+	Erythema with papules
2+	Edematous or vesicular reaction
3+	Spreading bullous or ulcerative reaction

REMOVAL OF THE PATCHES

Patches are removed approximately 48 hours after application. Most investigators remove the patches in the office, marking the sites in some fashion (Fig. 3–8). A fluorescent ink "highlighter"-type marking pen is useful for this purpose. When the patient returns for a later reading, the fluorescent ink is clearly visible under ultraviolet (Wood's lamp) light but is relatively invisible to the unaided eye. This is more aesthetically acceptable to the patient and less damaging to clothing than regular marking ink. With the new True-Test patches, the edge only may be marked and a plastic template used to determine patch position (Figs. 3–9 and 3–10).

READING PATCH TESTS

A preliminary testing is made at the time of removal of the patches. The NACDG grading system is listed in Table 3–1 (Figs. 3–11 to 3–14).

It cannot be overemphasized that a later reading after 48 hours is essential for accurate interpretation of patch test results. The most common interval for later reading is 72 hours (1 day after patch removal). A 96-hour reading is done by some investigators. At times, these readings are further supplemented with a final reading 1 week after patches are placed. The primary reason for the later readings is that a significant percentage of late positive test results are negative or questionable at the time of removal. Neomycin reactions, for instance, frequently fall in this category. In addition, as noted below, a later reading compared with the first reading may help differentiate an irritant from an allergic reaction. The added inconvenience to the patient or physician is far outweighed by the benefit of an accurate test result, either positive or negative.

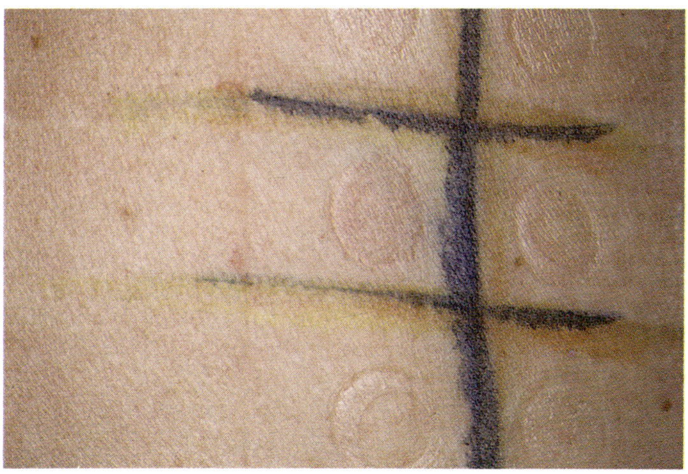

Figure 3–11 Questionable reaction, grade "?".

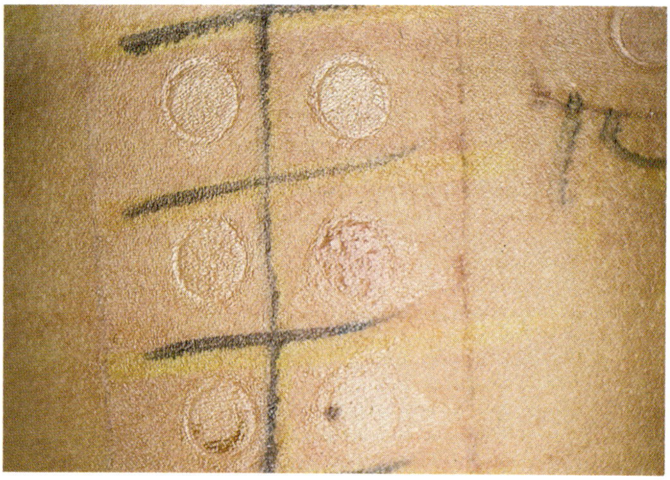

Figure 3–12 Positive reaction, grade "1."

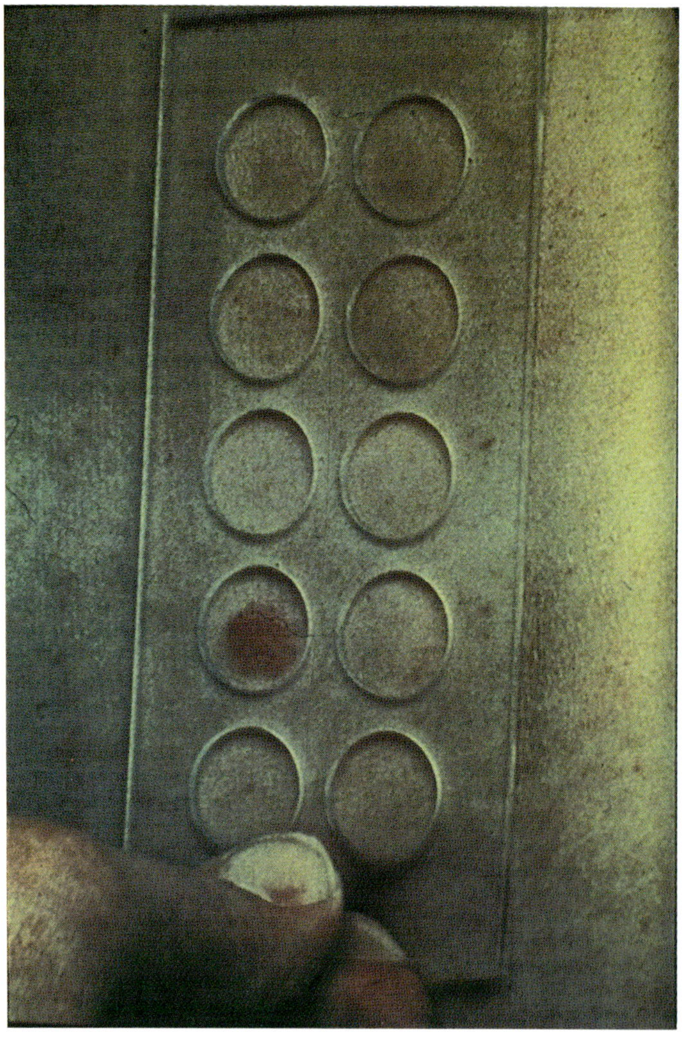

Figure 3–13 Strong positive reaction, grade "2."

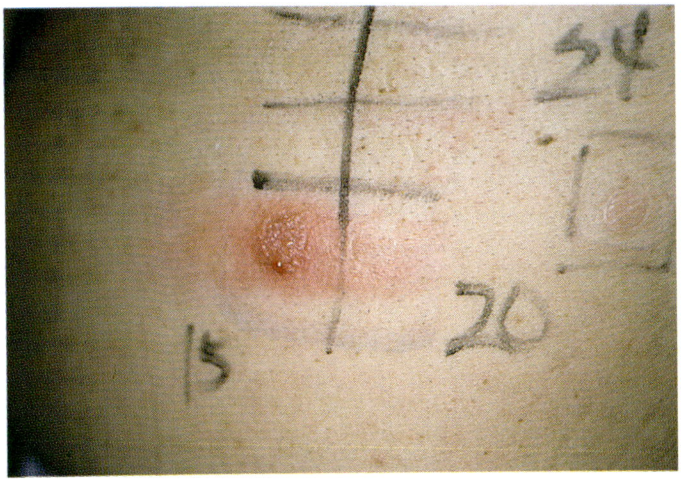

Figure 3–14 Extreme positive reaction, grade "3."

A false-positive irritant reaction may result from direct cutaneous toxicity rather than from an allergic response (Fig. 3–15). Although rare with standardized allergens, irritant reactions commonly occur when using patient-supplied items. Soaps and detergents, for instance, cause chemical damage to the epidermis and almost always produce an irritant reaction unless highly diluted before application. Irritant reactions usually do not spread from the test site and typically decrease in intensity from the earlier to the later reading. They may also show a blister with epidermal sloughing, suggesting a chemical burn.

In addition to irritant reactions, "excited skin" syndrome (or "angry back" syndrome) may cause false-positive test results (Fig. 3–16). This generalized state of cutaneous hyperreactivity usually occurs in a patient with active uncontrolled dermatitis at the time of testing and should be suspected when-

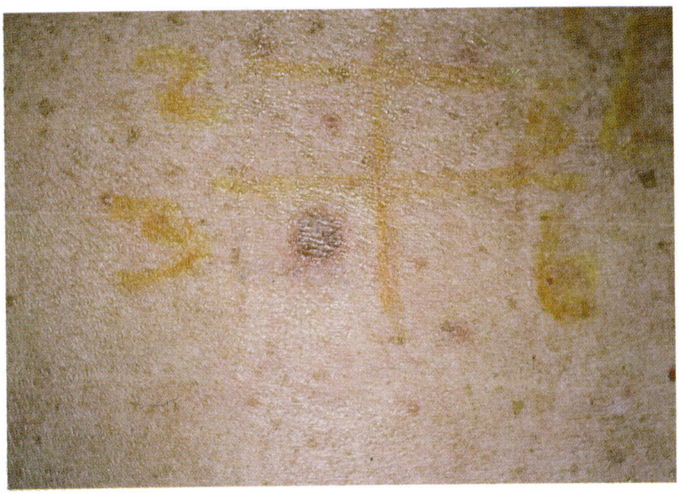

Figure 3–15 Probable irritant reaction.

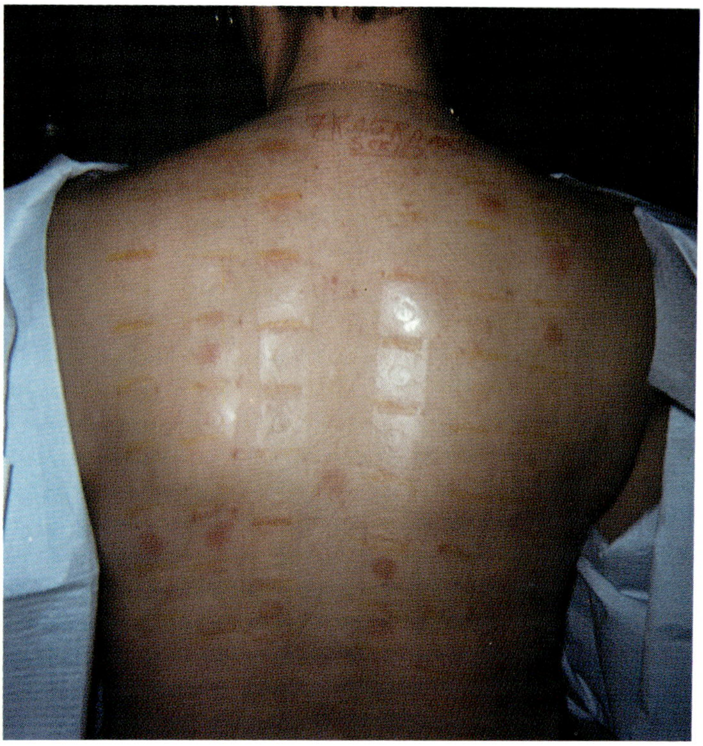

Figure 3–16 "Angry back" syndrome.

ever more than 10% of applied tests give positive results. If this occurs, the allergens showing a positive reaction should be retested, a few at a time, no sooner than 1 month after the original test. The patient should be free of active dermatitis. Usually, any positive reactions at this time are true, significant positives.

CONCLUSIONS

Proper patch-testing technique and interpretation, like all medical procedures, require skill and practice. Following the guidelines and recommendations given here will enhance the probability of significant, accurate results. The True-Test kit offers the advantage of ease of application with no preparation. True-Test is approved for sale in the United States. The twenty-item "standard" tray is also available commercially (from Hermal Company; see Appendix). Preparation and placement of the tests can usually be accomplished in an average of 10 to 15 minutes using the Finn Chambers technique and in several minutes using the True-Test kit.

ATLAS

Section I

Routine Screening

ETHYLENEDIAMINE HYDROCHLORIDE

HISTORY

This man has had a long-standing dermatitis that improved with topical and systemic corticosteroid therapy but failed to heal. When questioned about drug therapy, he specifically denied using anything other than that prescribed by his referring physician. Because of dermatitis chronicity, he was patch tested with the routine test series.

He had one positive reaction that appeared relevant—ethylenediamine hydrochloride. This ingredient was present in a tube of Mycolog cream that he had used.

RESOLUTION

On discontinuing use of Mycolog cream, his condition gradually improved and there has been no recurrence.

CLINICAL COMMENTS

Iatrogenic dermatitis due to Mycolog was brought to our attention by the late Otis Jillson. After he reported several patients from New Hampshire, it quickly became apparent that there were similar patients throughout the United States. The frequency of ethylenediamine hypersensitivity in an eczema population was subsequently found to be in excess of 5%. Concern in the dermatologic community about this led the manufacturers to reformulate Mycolog, removing ethylenediamine from the product. The result is Mycolog II. Several generic imitators of Mycolog cream are now available. Most of these contain ethylenediamine hydrochloride. It is important to remember that Mycolog *ointment* does not contain this stabilizer.

Some positive reactions to ethylenediamine cannot be traced to their source. Many occupational sources of ethylenediamine exist, but the relationship of the occupational exposure to unexplained reactions often remains unknown.

Ethylenediamine is released from aminophylline. For this reason, ethylenediamine-sensitive patients should not receive aminophylline, except when absolutely necessary, and then only when under close medical supervision.

The ethylenediamine class of antihistamines may produce orally elicited systemic allergic contact dermatitis. These include hydroxyzine, tripelennamine, pyrilamine, and methapyrilene.

Reference

Provost TT, Jillson OF: Ethylenediamine contact dermatitis. Arch Dermatol 96:231, 1967.

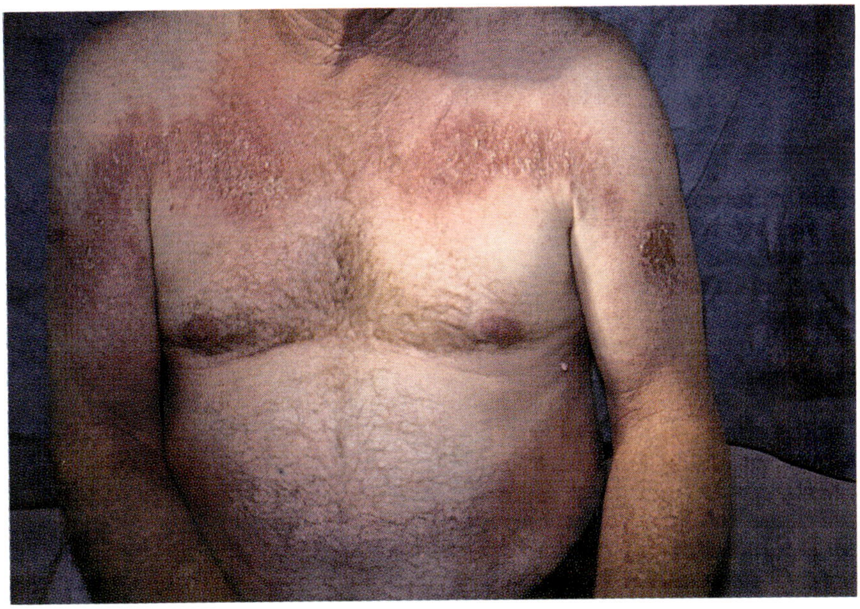

ETHYLENEDIAMINE

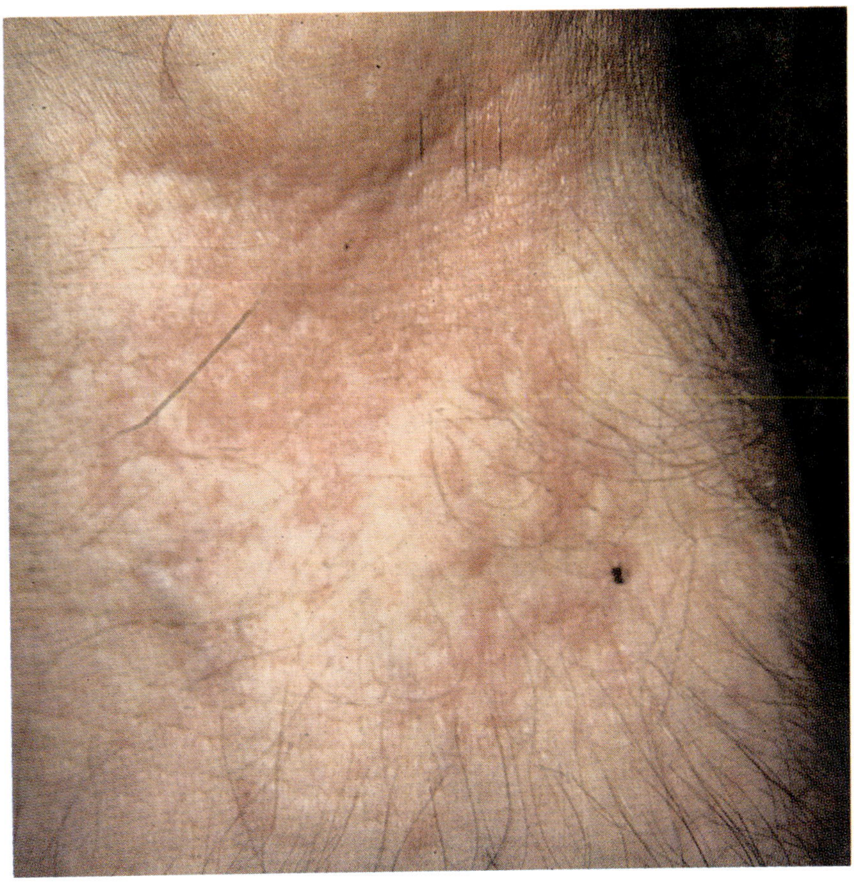

ETHYLENEDIAMINE

LANOLIN ALCOHOL (WOOL WAX ALCOHOL)

HISTORY

This woman, otherwise in good health, had chronic stasis dermatitis. Consultation with two dermatologists failed to produce healing. Several courses of topical and systemic corticoids were beneficial; nevertheless, the process was one of corticoid-induced remission followed by exacerbation with corticoid discontinuation.

RESOLUTION

Because of the chronic nature of her dermatitis, she was patch tested with the routine test series and her skin care products as well. The results showed strong positive reactions to wool wax alcohol and a commercial skin moisturizing cream manufactured by a major cosmetic firm. Identification of the allergen, present in the moisturizing cream, and instruction in inspecting the labels of skin care products resulted in gradual and complete healing of the dermatitis.

CLINICAL COMMENTS

Wool wax alcohol is synonymous with lanolin alcohol. In spite of decades of intense chemical and clinical study, the allergen in lanolin remains elusive. Current studies suggest the allergen fractionates with the wool wax alcohol fraction.

Lanolin is not a pure substance; patch testing is characteristically performed with high concentrations of lanolin (20% wool wax alcohol in petrolatum). In spite of this, not all lanolin-sensitive people react to the standard test series for wool wax alcohol. For that reason, when clinically indicated, the lanolin the patient uses also should be tested.

Wool wax alcohol is a marginal irritant in some individuals. Weak positive results may reveal sensitization or irritation. When in doubt, a provocative use test or repeat open application test is indicated.

The most common source of lanolin sensitivity in the United States is lanolin used in the treatment of leg ulcers. It has been suggested that lanolin can be tolerated by lanolin-sensitive people when it is applied to normal skin, although this is not always the case.

Reference

Cronin E: Lanolin dermatitis. Br J Dermatol 78:617, 1966.

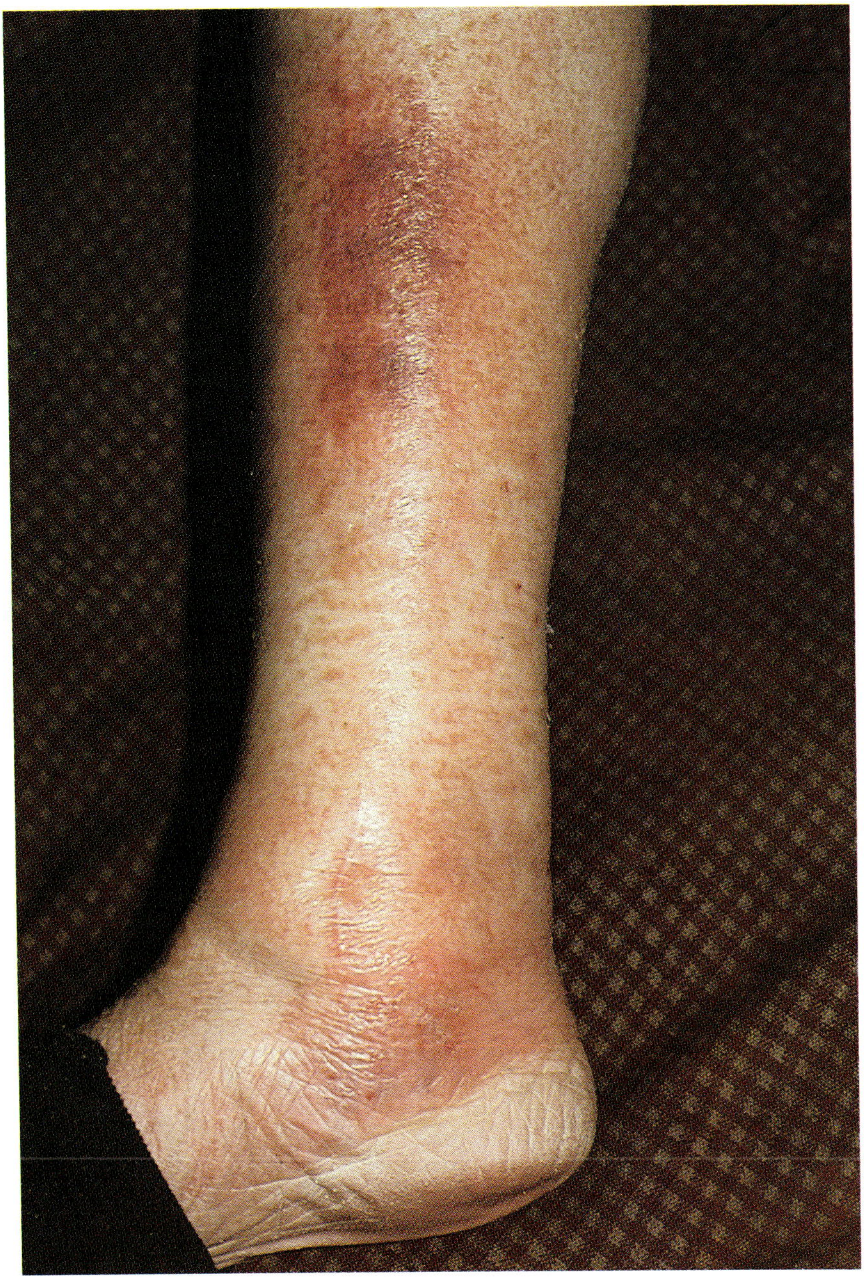

LANOLIN ALCOHOL (WOOL WAX ALCOHOL)

BENZOCAINE

CASE I

History

This patient with a recurring chronic hand eczema for several years returned to the dermatologist because of an exacerbation (*A*). Routine patch testing, including the routine test series and the patient's medicaments and gloves, revealed a presumably relevant allergen—benzocaine.

Resolution

With benzocaine discontinuation, the dermatitis resolved. The patient was instructed to read labels on products for benzocaine content and also about the possibility of cross reactions to closely related materials such as paraphenylenediamine.

CASE II

History

This patient had chronic perirectal itching (*B*). The patient sought relief from a pharmacist by obtaining a medication containing a local anesthetic.

Resolution

Patch testing with the offending formulation and benzocaine in petrolatum revealed positive reactions. The condition cleared rapidly when the benzocaine formulation was discontinued.

CLINICAL COMMENTS

Benzocaine sensitivity is relatively uncommon, in spite of its reputation to the contrary. In an epidemiologic study in normal subjects in San Francisco, approximately one in 1000 volunteers was found to be sensitized. In aimed patch testing in eczema patients in 1990, approximately 2% of patients studied by the North American Contact Dermatitis Research Group were patch test positive.

It is important to remember that benzocaine cross reacts with many "para"-substances such as paraphenylenediamine.

The patient should receive instructions regarding the difference between benzocaine and certain other chemically unrelated "caines," such as lidocaine, which can be safely used. Because patients often have difficulty remembering medicament sensitivity, it is appropriate to provide an instruction card for the patient's wallet or purse.

References

Fisher AA: Contact Dermatitis, 3rd ed. Philadelphia, Lea & Febiger, 1986, pp 220–223.
Prystowsky SD, et al: Allergic contact hypersensitivity to nickel, neomycin, ethylenediamine and benzocaine. Arch Dermatol 115:959 1979.

A

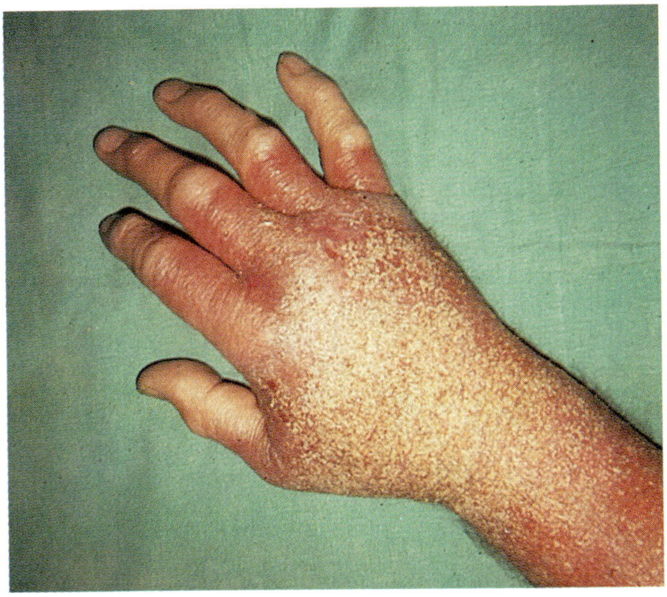

Courtesy of Frances J. Storrs, M.D.

BENZOCAINE

B

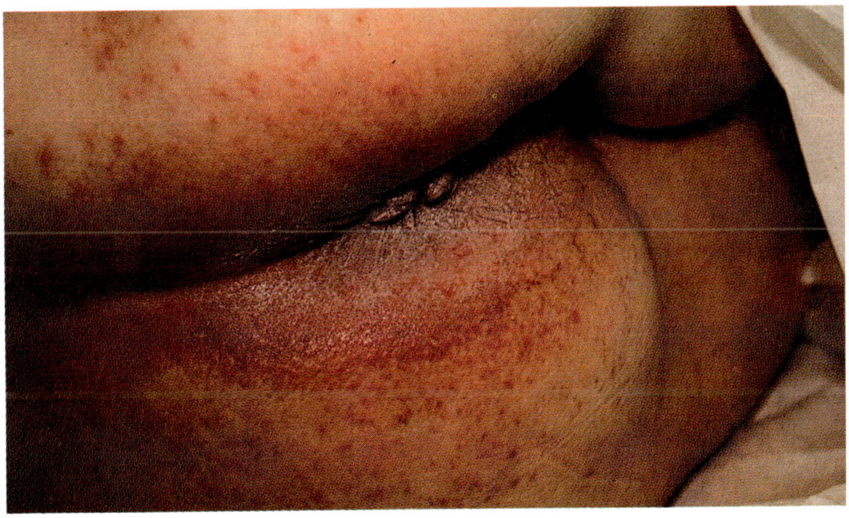

BENZOCAINE

QUATERNIUM-15

HISTORY

This woman has had a long-standing indolent dermatitis, generally chronic but partially responsive to topical corticosteroids. Patch testing with the routine series revealed a strong positive reaction to Quaternium-15.

RESOLUTION

The condition cleared completely when the patient began to identify Quaternium-15 on labels, and discontinued use of Quaternium-15–containing products.

CLINICAL COMMENTS

Quaternium-15 is a widely used biocide, appearing in skin care products, cosmetics, dermatologics, and industry. Under appropriate circumstances it releases formaldehyde and is not water-stable. Quaternium-15–sensitive patients may or may not be formalin-sensitive also. Quaternium-15–sensitive patients may tolerate Quaternium-15–preserved products, presumably because their level of use application is lower than their patch test sensitivity. Nevertheless, as a general rule, we recommend that patients identify Quaternium-15 on labels and avoid the use of Quaternium-15 products until the dermatitis is healed, plus a minimum of a 3-month waiting period. Since Quaternium-15 releases formaldehyde, patients may also react to other formaldehyde releasers such as imidazolidinyl urea. This picture shows the typical blotchy appearance.

Reference

Fransway AF: The problem of preservation in the 1990's: I. Statement of the problem, solution(s) of the industry, and the current use of formaldehyde and formaldehyde-releasing biocides. Am J Cont Dermatol 2:6–23, 1991.

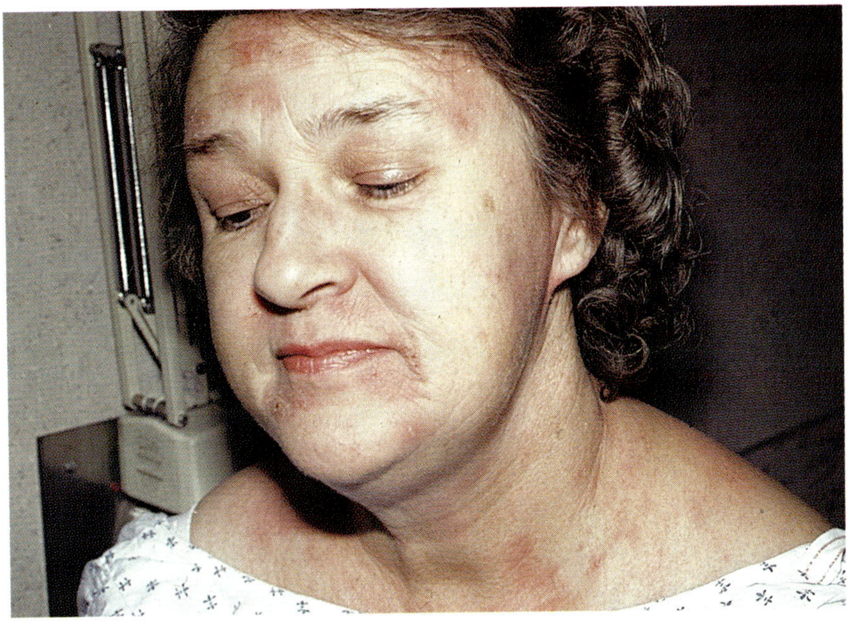

Courtesy of Frances J. Storrs, M.D.

QUATERNIUM-15

IMIDAZOLIDINYL UREA

HISTORY

This woman has had multiple episodes of facial dermatitis, usually responsive to topical corticosteroids. Because of chronicity, the patient was patch tested with the routine series, to fragrances, to preservatives, and to her facial care products. Tests showed strong reactions to imidazolidinyl urea and formalin.

RESOLUTION

The condition rapidly cleared when the patient learned to identify this preservative and to avoid it.

CLINICAL COMMENTS

Because imidazolidinyl urea is a formaldehyde releaser, the patient may be patch test sensitive to the preservative alone or to the preservative and formaldehyde. As with other formaldehyde releasers, not all patients who are patch test positive are clinically intolerant when the material is applied to normal skin. They may react to other formaldehyde releasers, presumably because of the formaldehyde release. This biocide is currently an ingredient in numerous skin care products, dermatologics, and cosmetics.

Reference

Fransway AF: The problem of preservation in the 1990's: I. Statement of the problem, solution(s) of the industry, and the current use of formaldehyde and formaldehyde-releasing biocides. Am J Cont Dermatol 2:6–23, 1991.

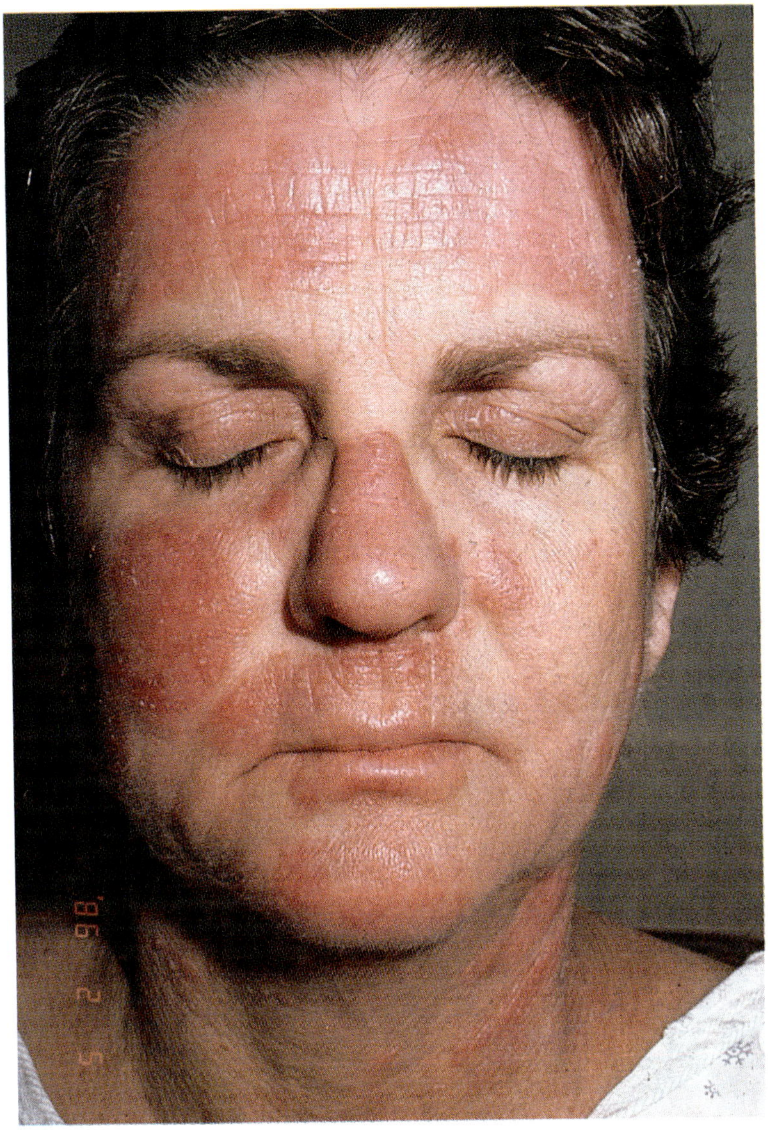

Courtesy of Frances J. Storrs, M.D.

IMIDAZOLIDINYL UREA

BALSAM OF PERU

HISTORY

This child was being treated for a nonspecific eczematous eruption with vitamin A&D ointment. Patch testing with the ointment was positive. Testing with the components revealed a positive reaction to balsam of Peru.

RESOLUTION

The condition cleared completely when the child avoided use of the product.

CLINICAL COMMENT

Balsam of Peru is a natural material derived from the tree *Myroxolon balsamum*. This tree grows in San Salvador and is present in many other parts of the world; it is common to mix balsams from several countries for manufacture of antigens for diagnostic purposes.

The material is a natural product and is not reproducible from batch to batch. It is an efficient marker for fragrance sensitivity, with approximately one-half of people with known fragrance allergy reacting to it. It contains many well-known allergens: a partial listing includes cinnamic acid, benzyl alcohol, vanillin, and others. Isoeugenol, eugenol, orange peel, and clove often show cross reactions with balsam of Peru. Balsam of Peru and cinnamic aldehyde also produce nonimmunologic contact urticaria. The balsam is both a fragrance material and a wound-healing agent and also has antimicrobial properties.

Occasionally, it may be a marker for orally elicited allergic contact dermatitis, as shown by Hjorth in his monograph. To demonstrate this, the patient ingests flavorings such as cinnamon and rapidly develops a flare of dermatitis from this oral exposure.

Sensitization to balsam of Peru may produce dermatitis in dentists, bakers, food handlers, beekeepers, and laboratory technicians.

References

Fisher AA: Contact Dermatitis, 3rd ed. Philadelphia, Lea & Febiger, 1986, pp 422–424.
Hjorth N: Eczematous Allergy to Balsams, Allied Perfumes, and Flavoring Agents. Copenhagen, Munksgaard, 1961.

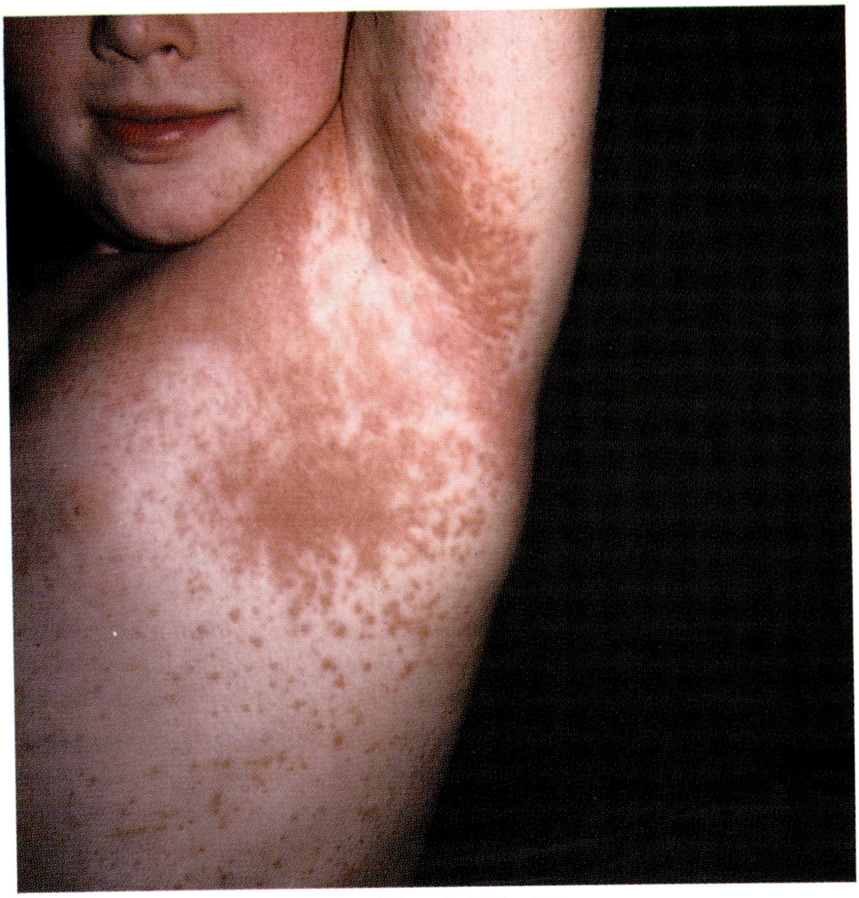

Courtesy of Alexander A. Fisher, M.D.

BALSAM OF PERU

CINNAMIC ALDEHYDE (CINNAMAL)

HISTORY

This young woman had used axillary products for years without difficulty. Recently, she developed an eruption. Patch testing with her deodorant gave a positive reaction. Subsequent testing with a fragrance test series revealed a strong reaction to 1% cinnamic aldehyde in petrolatum. The manufacturer confirmed the presence of cinnamic aldehyde in the fragrance of this axillary product but did not disclose its concentration.

RESOLUTION

The condition subsequently cleared spontaneously, upon cessation of product use. In the future, she should use an unscented deodorant or, prior to use of a scented deodorant, do a repeat open application test in the antecubital fossa.

CLINICAL COMMENTS

Cinnamic aldehyde (cinnamaldehyde, cinnamal) is one of the most common fragrance allergens in those studies in which the fragrance breakdowns were defined. One must be cautious in emphasizing in such a statement that all fragrance materials have been tested.

The axilla is an anatomic site that seems, at least in theory, to be especially likely to develop sensitization. This is based upon the fact that it is anatomically occlusive and hence would lend itself to increased penetration. We do not have epidemiologic data to determine whether biologically this is, in fact, the case.

Cinnamic aldehyde is converted by the skin's enzymes into cinnamic alcohol (cinnamyl alcohol), another fragrance and flavoring agent. Many patients who are cinnamic aldehyde- or alcohol-positive react to balsam of Peru, a natural mixture. This is not surprising in that the balsam contains many cinnamic derivatives. In some countries, the second screening material for fragrance after balsam of Peru is the fragrance mix; cinnamic aldehyde is in all of the currently used diagnostic fragrance mixtures.

Numerous examples of orally elicited allergic contact dermatitis caused by cinnamic aldehyde have been documented. This is due to the fact that many flavoring agents (e.g., cinnamon) contain cinnamic aldehyde.

Cinnamic aldehyde is a marginal irritant at a concentration of 1% in petrolatum. When there is doubt, a provocative use test or repeat open application test with the allergen itself will be confirmatory.

As with all contact allergens, there is a dose-response curve. The patient may be able to tolerate those fragranced formulations in which cinnamic aldehyde or alcohol is present at extremely low levels. This is especially true of wash-off products such as shampoos and bar soaps. Because of this aspect of a dose-response curve, and because of regional variation in proclivity to allergic contact dermatitis, we often recommend that the patient do a provocative use test with fragranced products approximately 6 to 9 months after the dermatitis has completely cleared. This is a suitable way for fragrance-sensitive patients to identify which products they can safely use. When more complete fragrance ingredient label disclosure becomes a reality (as is the case with cosmetic ingredients in many countries), the patient will be able to make a more informed choice of product.

References

Larsen WG: Perfume dermatitis. J Am Acad Dermatol 12:1–9, 1985.
Larsen WG: How to instruct patients sensitive to fragrances. J Am Acad Dermatol 21:880, 1989.
Weibel H, Hansen J: Penetration of the fragrance compounds, cinnamaldehyde and cinnamyl alcohol, through human skin in vitro. Contact Dermatitis 20:167–172, 1989.

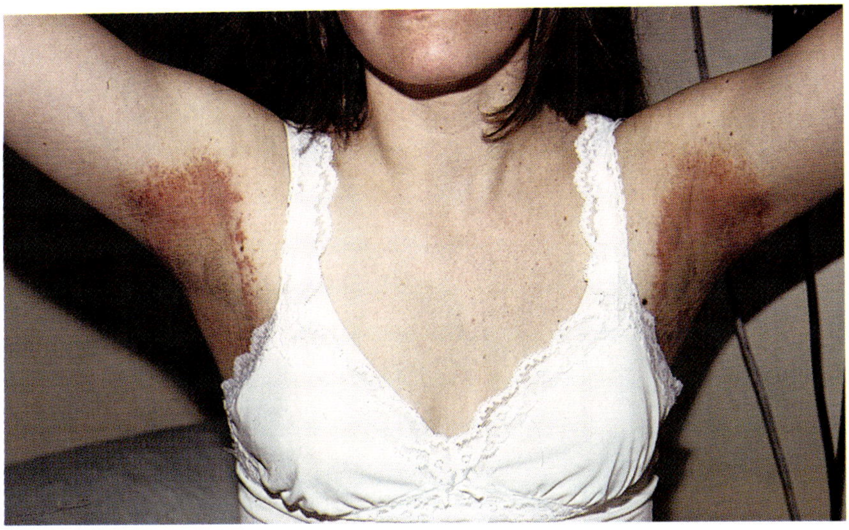

CINNAMIC ALDEHYDE (CINNAMAL)

HEXAVALENT CHROMIUM

HISTORY

This 57-year-old cement worker developed a generalized, highly pruritic, exudative dermatitis in all exposed areas, particularly the hands, arms, neck, face, and the legs at the boot tops. He had had a recurring, usually mild, hand dermatitis for many years (*A*).

Another man developed dermatitis on the buttocks beneath the pocket where he carried his leather wallet (*B*).

RESOLUTION

To eliminate hexavalent chromium from cement by chemical reduction, several countries, including Poland and Denmark, utilize the method of Fregert and associates of adding iron sulfate to the cement during mixing. In a recent Danish study, this method appears to have significantly decreased the number of new patients sensitized to hexavalent chromium.

In the United States, for reasons not completely explained, chromium sensitization due to cement appears to be decreasing. Cement dermatitis due to chromium is often chronic. Nevertheless, many cement workers, although sensitized, can continue to work. Details are found in the monograph of Høvding. Furthermore, even when a chromium-sensitized cement worker is removed from work, the dermatitis may persist. The reasons for this are not understood.

CLINICAL COMMENT

Although present in minute quantities, hexavalent chromium is the chief allergen in cement. The frequency of sensitization is related to the concentration of chromium and the closeness of skin contact. The marked alkalinity of cement is believed to be an important predisposing factor.

Potassium dichromate is tested in the United States at a concentration of 0.25% and in other countries at a concentration of 0.5%. Using either concentration, a significant number of weak positive reactions (questionable responses) result; these reactions are usually irritant in nature. When in doubt, a repeat patch test should be done. Rarely, it is necessary to do intradermal testing to confirm the presence of allergic contact sensitization.

Other uses of chromium include the tanning of leather, rust inhibition in paints and other substances, and as an oxidizing agent in chemicals, dyes, and intermediates. It is also present in certain photographic materials, among numerous other uses.

References

Adams RM: Occupational Skin Disease, 2nd ed. Philadelphia, Saunders, 1990, pp 353–364.

Burrows D: Chromium: Metabolism and Toxicity. Boca Raton, FL, CRC Press, 1983.

Fregert S, Gruvberger B, Sandahl E: Reduction of chromate in cement by iron sulfate. Contact Dermatitis 5:39–42, 1979.

Høvding G: Cement eczema and chromium allergy: An epidemiological investigation. Thesis. Bergen, Norway, University of Bergen, 1970.

A

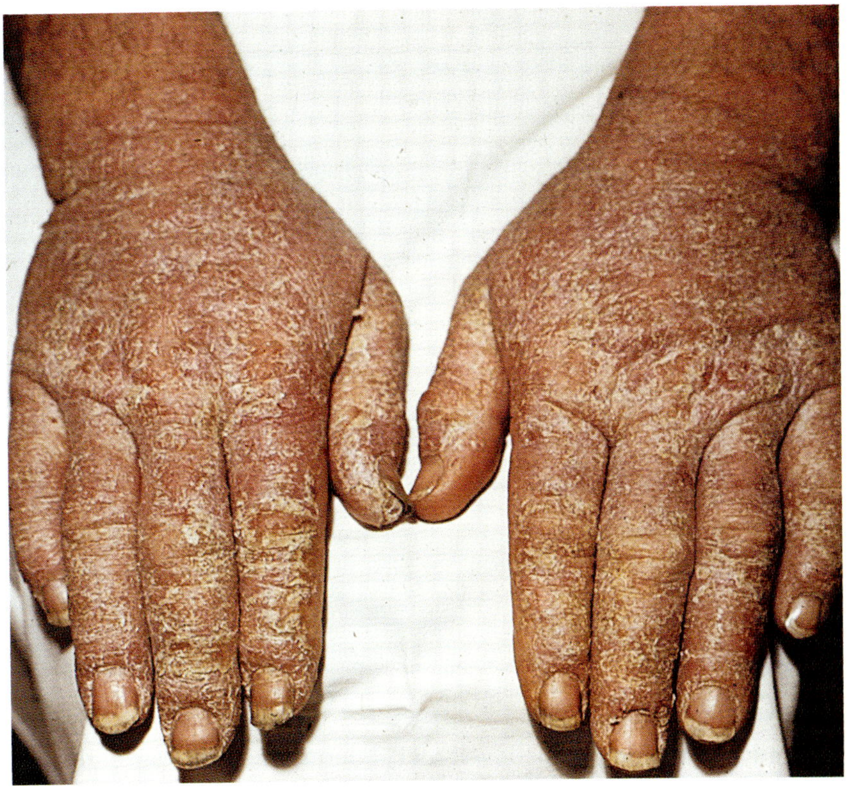

HEXAVALENT CHROMIUM

B

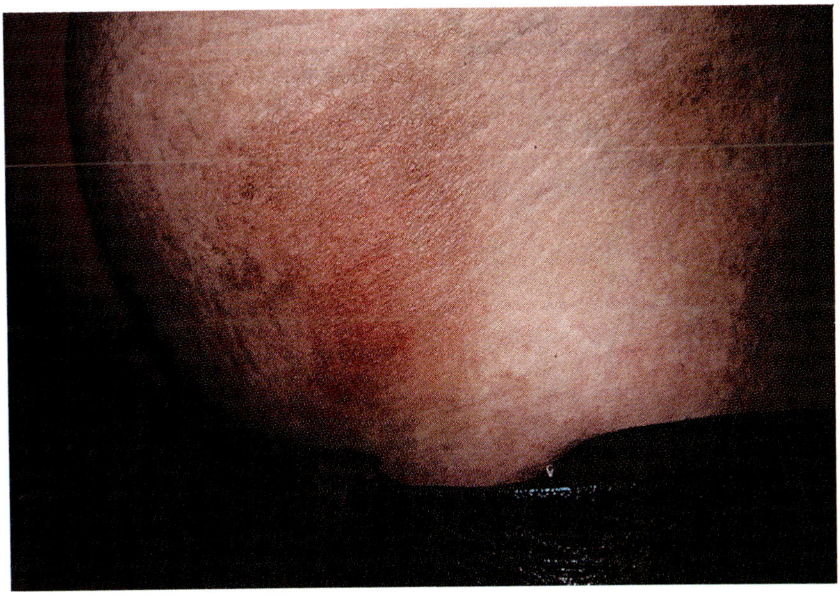

HEXAVALENT CHROMIUM

RUBBER

HISTORY

This nurse's duties included frequently taking blood pressure readings (*A*). Her dermatitis improved somewhat on weekends and during periods away from work but regularly recurred within a day or two of returning to work. The dermatitis was worse on the right palm.

A 52-year-old tombstone maker was extremely sensitive to the rubber apron and gloves he regularly wore in his work (*B*). The routine testing was performed with a piece of his rubber apron.

A
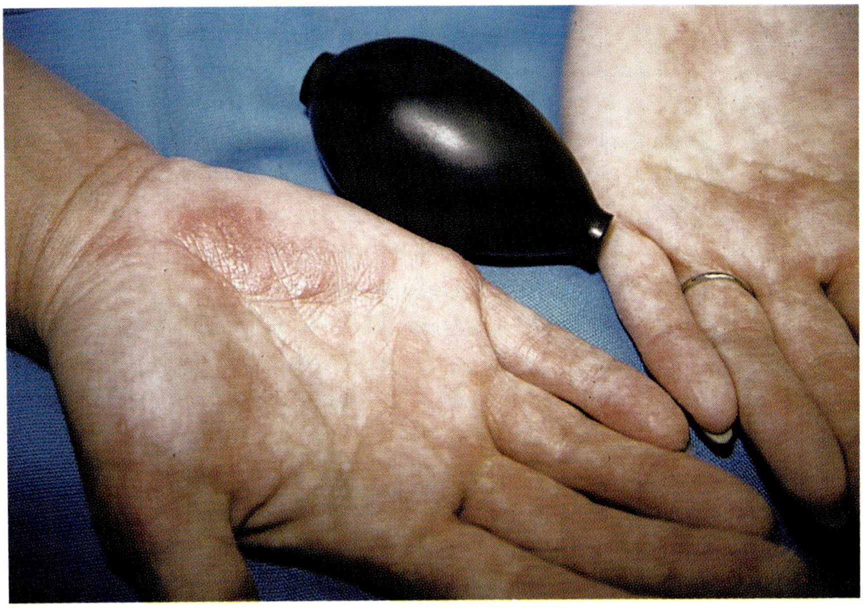

RUBBER

B
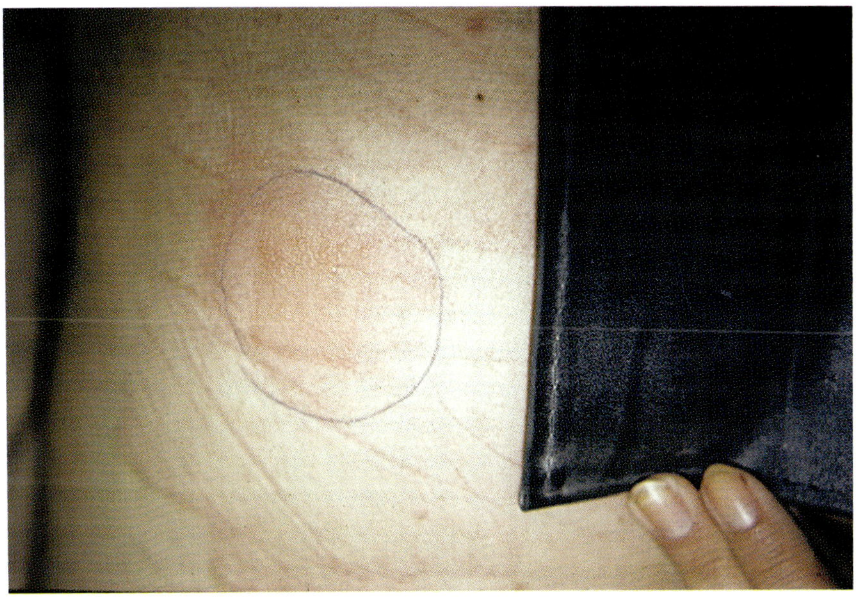

RUBBER

RUBBER *Continued*

This shows a 52-year-old housewife who is markedly sensitive to rubber household gloves (*C*).

A barber developed contact dermatitis from the rubber band on a hand-held scalp vibrator (*D*).

RESOLUTION

Patch testing is important to identify the specific allergens in rubber gloves because rubber that does not contain a particular chemical is often available. Household surgical and work gloves are available without the common contact allergens. For ordinary uses, polyvinyl-type gloves are suitable for those allergic to rubber chemicals.

CLINICAL COMMENTS

Rubber allergy is a common condition seen in dermatologists' offices. The two most frequent allergens in rubber are mercaptobenzothiazole and tetramethyl thiuram disulfide. Unlike many other substances, such as most plastics, rubber releases these allergens readily onto the skin, especially when the skin is occluded and perspiring.

The rubber chemicals currently available in the routine testing series do not include every rubber allergen. Thus, it is important to test all patients with hand dermatitis with their own gloves; this is because the morphology may be atypical. Some physicians prefer to use both sides of the gloves; if the outside tests positive and the inside negative, this suggests the possibility of an additional chemical other than that of the glove. Allergic contact dermatitis to natural, untreated latex does not occur. However, immediate-type sensitivity such as contact urticaria does. Delayed-type sensitization occurs from the additives, rather than from latex. With few exceptions, it is difficult or impossible to learn which additives are present in a given rubber product. Unfortunately, commercially available spot tests are presently unavailable.

Thiuram-sensitive patients may develop a generalized dermatitis following ingestion of Antabuse, used to treat alcoholism.

It is important to note that thiurams and the related carbamates are widely used as pesticides in agriculture.

References

Adams RM: Occupational Skin Disease, 2nd ed. Philadelphia, WB Saunders, 1990, pp 462–485.
Cronin E: Contact Dermatitis. New York, Churchill Livingstone, 1980, pp 714–770.
Fisher AA: Contact Dermatitis, 3rd ed. Philadelphia, Lea & Febiger, 1986, pp 603–643.

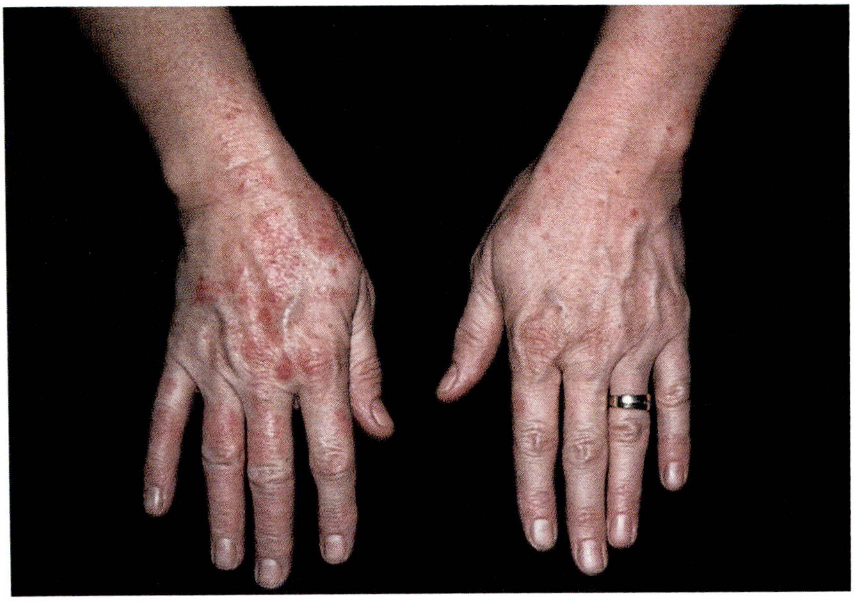

C

RUBBER

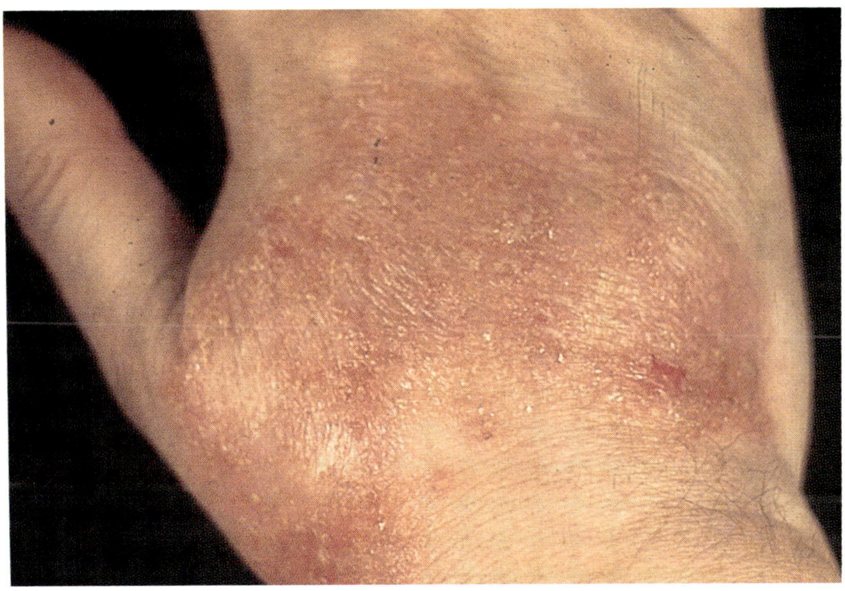

D

RUBBER

FORMALDEHYDE (FORMALIN)

HISTORY

This patient slowly developed a widespread dermatitis, especially involving the axillary folds and waist. The patient was treated for endogenous eczema for approximately 1 year. Subsequent patch testing to 1% formaldehyde in water revealed a 2+ reaction at 48 and 96 hours. On morphologic and clinical history grounds, this dermatitis may be easily confused with endogenous eczema and the so-called "baboon syndrome" (see p. 198).

RESOLUTION

A diagnosis of formalin clothing dermatitis was made and the patient instructed in the use of allergen alternatives.

CLINICAL COMMENTS

Formalin is ubiquitous. Fortunately, few people become sensitized because the amount of allergen is usually insufficient to either induce or elicit a clinical response.

Clothing dermatitis may be due to dyes (see p. 106), formaldehyde-based resins (see p. 108), or formaldehyde itself.

The patch test concentration depends upon the type of patch used in testing. When using the Al test, for example, the concentration is 2% in water, whereas in the Finn Chambers, it is 1% in water.

Formalin is widely used as a preservative, as in shampoos, for example. Biocides, which release formaldehyde, include Quaternium-15, imidazolidinyl urea (Germal I), and diazolidinyl urea (Germal II). Thus, it is very important to inform patients about the preservatives that are formaldehyde releasers.

Raw ingredients may be preserved with formalin, which is infrequently disclosed on labels.

Contact urticaria of the immunologic type has been demonstrated from formaldehyde.

Many formalin-sensitive patients can tolerate low levels of formaldehyde, as can be demonstrated by the careful use of a provocative use test or a repeat open application test.

Reference

Fransway AF: The problem of preservation in 1990's: Statement of the problem, solution(s) of the industry, and the current use of formaldehyde and formaldehyde-releasing biocides. Am J Cont Dermatol 2:6–23, 1991.

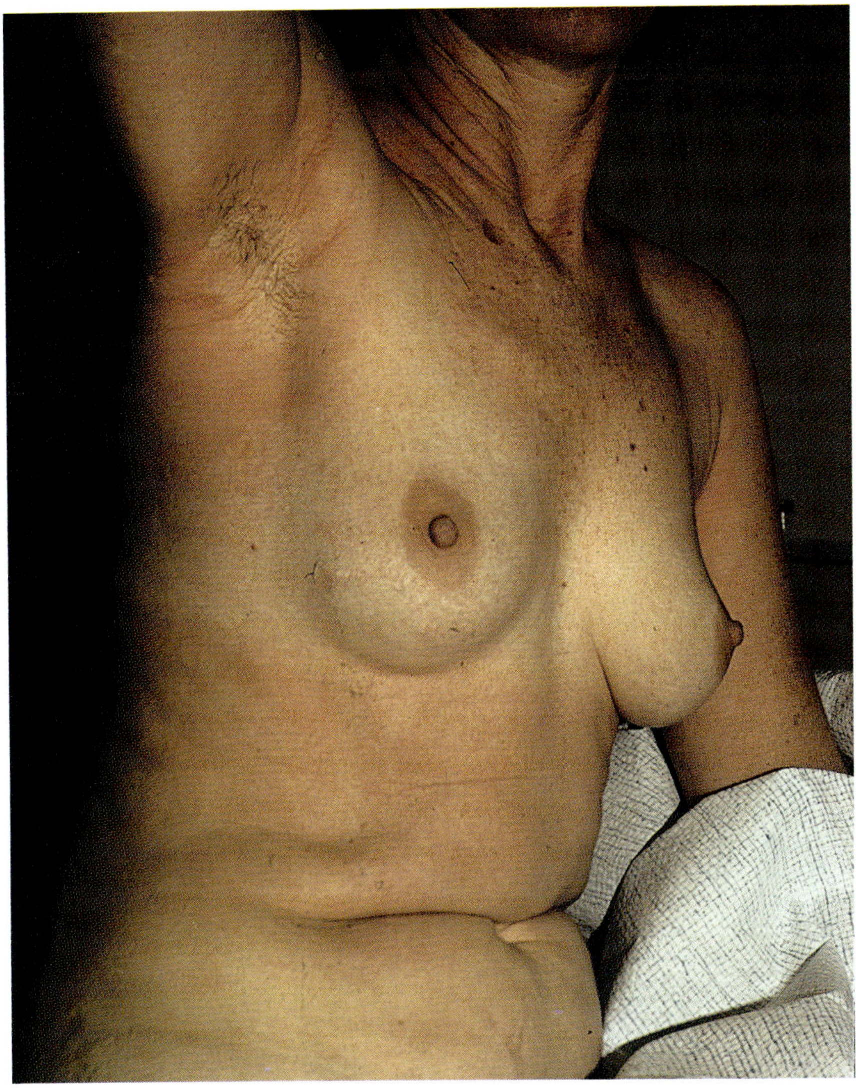

Courtesy of Alexander A. Fisher, M.D.

FORMALDEHYDE (FORMALIN)

PARAPHENYLENEDIAMINE

HISTORY

This young woman had dyed her hair for years without incident. Eighteen hours after the most recent hair dyeing, she developed marked eyelid swelling. The photograph shows the patient approximately 24 hours after hair dyeing.

RESOLUTION

Treatment consisted of systemic corticosteroids. Resolution was complete.

CLINICAL COMMENTS

Hair dye dermatitis usually spares the scalp to a large extent and instead involves the eyelids, forehead, ears, and neck. Occasionally, distant lesions may occur. Although it is considered an example of delayed hypersensitivity, many patients develop eyelid swelling rather rapidly, suggesting that immediate hypersensitivity may be part of the pathophysiology.

Diagnosis is made on the basis of history, morphology, and patch testing. Most patients make the diagnosis themselves; in some instances, it is covert and requires considerable sleuthing on the part of the physician. In these cases, the patients do not relate the dermatitis to the use of the hair tint.

For diagnostic patch testing, 1% paraphenylenediamine in petrolatum is used. Some patients with hair dye dermatitis are *not* sensitized to paraphenylenediamine and should be tested with the components as well as the hair dye itself.

Manufacturers of hair tints have long recommended open testing, retroauricularly, to the undiluted final product. It seems likely that most consumers and beauticians disregard this.

Open testing should be done at the same time as patch testing to identify that the product is, in fact, the cause. In addition, ingredient testing is always required to find the specific allergen and recommend an alternative. For instance, when resorcinol is the allergen (albeit rarely), resorcinol-free formulations are available.

Semipermanent hair dyes are commonly recommended when permanent dyes produce sensitization. Semipermanent hair dyes contain *substituted* paraphenylenediamines (e.g., nitro-p-phenylenediamine) and may be as allergenic as paraphenylenediamine and its derivatives found in permanent dyes.

A trial of semipermanent dyes should be done with medical supervision. The beautician must be especially cautious to minimize skin exposure, and a physician should be available to promptly treat the dermatitis if it develops.

Temporary tints and henna do not contain paraphenylenediamine, substituted paraphenylenediamines, or related substances, and they usually may be used without difficulty.

References

Adams RM: Occupational Skin Disease, 2nd ed. Philadelphia, WB Saunders, 1990, pp 340–342.

Engasser PG, Maibach HI: Cosmetics and dermatology: Hair dye toxicology. In Rook AJ, Maibach HI (eds.): Recent Advances in Dermatology 6. New York, Churchill Livingstone, 1985.

Fisher AA: Contact Dermatitis, 3rd ed. Philadelphia, Lea & Febiger, 1986, pp 380–382.

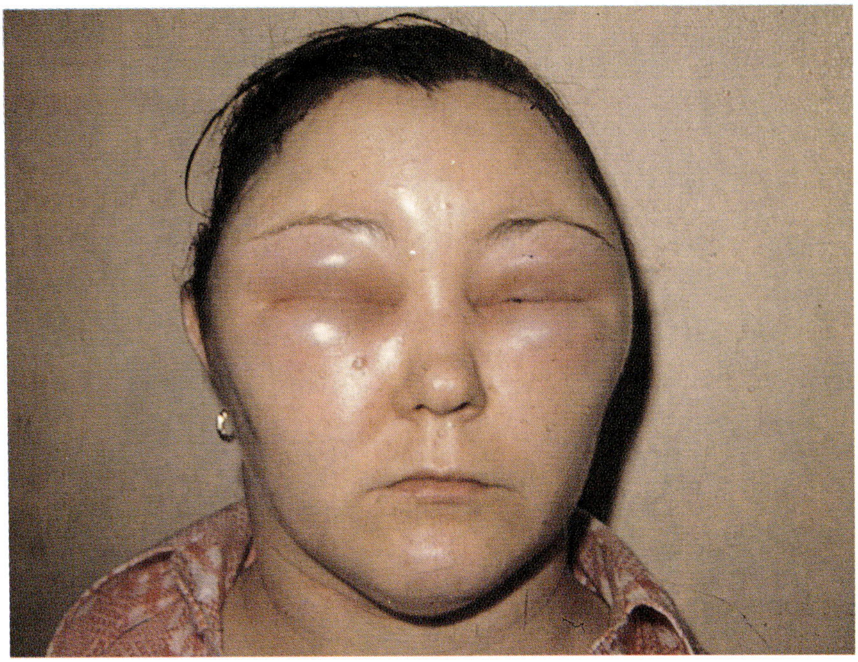

PARAPHENYLENEDIAMINE

EPOXY RESIN

HISTORY

This 24-year-old home hobbiest woodworker had used epoxy resins as adhesives for several years. He suddenly developed a highly pruritic dermatitis on the dorsum of his hand.

RESOLUTION

Treatment consisted of wet dressings and systemic corticosteroids.

CLINICAL COMMENTS

Epoxy resin dermatitis infrequently presents diagnostic difficulties in the workplace, because it is an overt allergen in industry. It appears that the allergen usually resides in the epoxy molecule. In recent years, as epoxy has become available for use in the home, increasing numbers of patients are seen in which it is a covert allergen. In these cases, routine battery testing produces a diagnosis that could otherwise have been unsuspected.

The allergen is often the epoxy itself. When testing with epoxy resin, the routine test series epoxy (molecular weight 340) will discern perhaps 80 to 90% of all epoxy allergy. Epoxy allergen chemistry is complex and varied; thus, individual patients, mainly those in industry, must be tested with the industrial epoxy actually used. Epoxy sensitization is almost always due to the low molecular weight types; those of higher molecular weight ($>$1000) are much less likely to sensitize skin.

Epoxy hardeners also must be considered as possible sensitizers. Industrial hardeners are not often present in the routine testing series available in most countries. Thus, it is important to obtain the actual hardener used by the patient and test at an appropriate, nonirritating concentration as suggested in standard textbooks.

Many products contain epoxy resins, and their presence would be otherwise unsuspected. Hearing aids, colored labels, and other common items are protected by epoxy resins, and they occasionally induce dermatitis. In women, except for those with occupational exposures, it is sometimes impossible to identify a source of exposure.

References

Adams RM: Occupational Skin Disease, 2nd ed. Philadelphia, WB Saunders, 1990, pp 387–407.
Fisher AA: Contact Dermatitis, 3rd ed. Philadelphia, Lea & Febiger, 1986, pp 549–554.
Malten K: Industrial Toxicology and Dermatology in the Production and Processing of Plastics. New York, Elsevier Publishing, 1964.

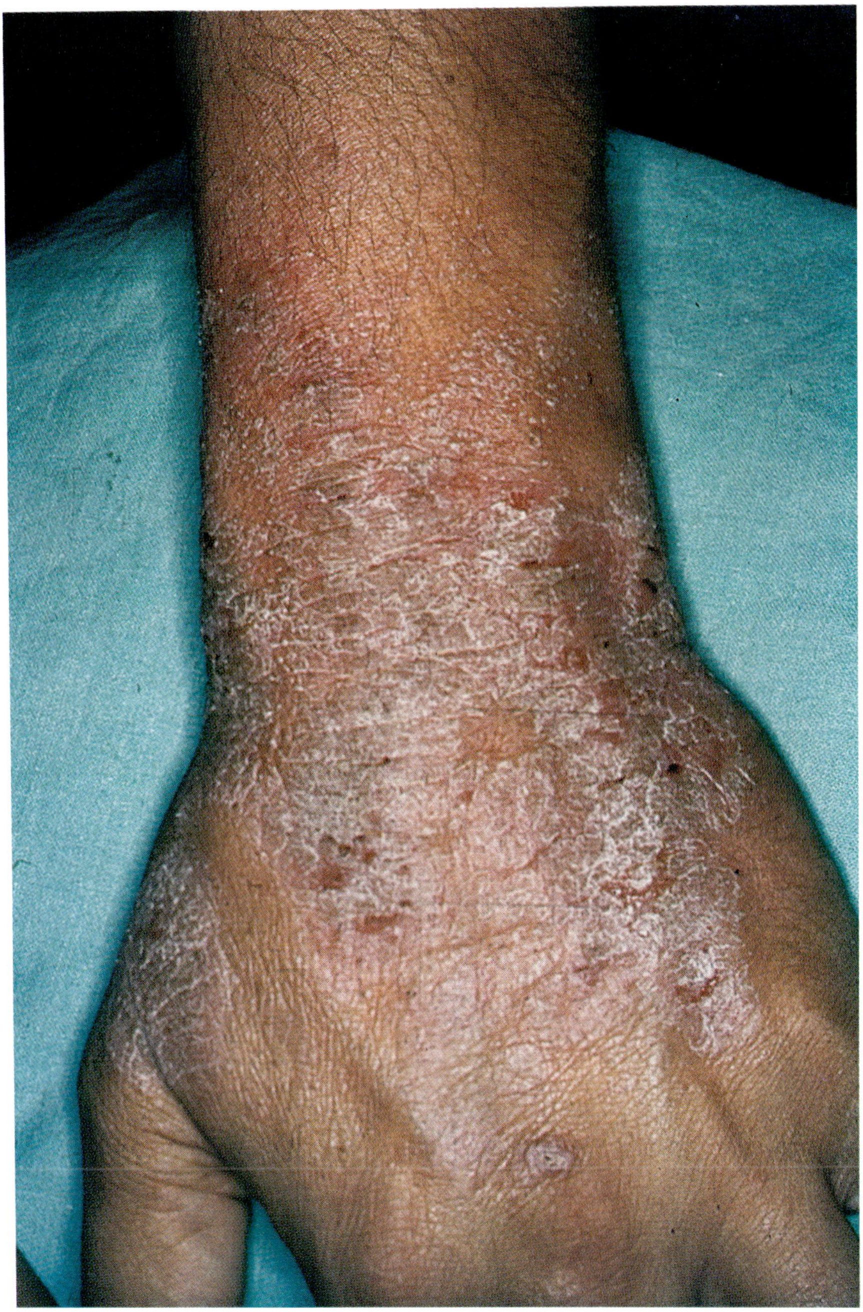

Courtesy of Alexander A. Fisher, M.D.

EPOXY RESIN

PARATERTIARY BUTYLPHENOL FORMALDEHYDE RESIN

HISTORY

This young man developed a dermatitis beneath the key case he carried in his trouser pocket (*A*). The dermatitis was highly pruritic and erythematous with some blistering.

This woman had worn a leather watchband for many years. Several days after purchasing a new one, a pruritic dermatitis appeared (*B*).

RESOLUTION

Both patients had rapid clearing of their dermatitis after establishing the cause and effect relationship and discontinuing contact. In the second patient, sensitization presumably had occurred earlier because of the rapid onset of dermatitis.

CLINICAL COMMENTS

This resin, utilized as an adhesive, is a highly complex synthetic material that varies from batch to batch and supplier to supplier. Much of our knowledge regarding sensitization comes from cases of industrial exposure; one must test patients not only with this material in the routine test series, but also with the specific resin employed in the workplace.

In nonoccupational exposure, the most common source of dermatitis is an adhesive used in shoe fabrication.

References

Adams RM: Occupational Skin Disease, 2nd ed. Philadelphia, WB Saunders, 1990, pp 402–403.
Bruze M: Contact sensitizers in resins based on phenol and formaldehyde. Thesis. Lund, Sweden, University of Lund, 1985.
Fisher AA: Contact Dermatitis, 3rd ed. Philadelphia, Lea & Febiger, 1986, pp 649–651.
Malten KE: Occupational eczema due to paratertiary butylphenol in a shoe adhesive. Dermatologica 117:103, 1958.

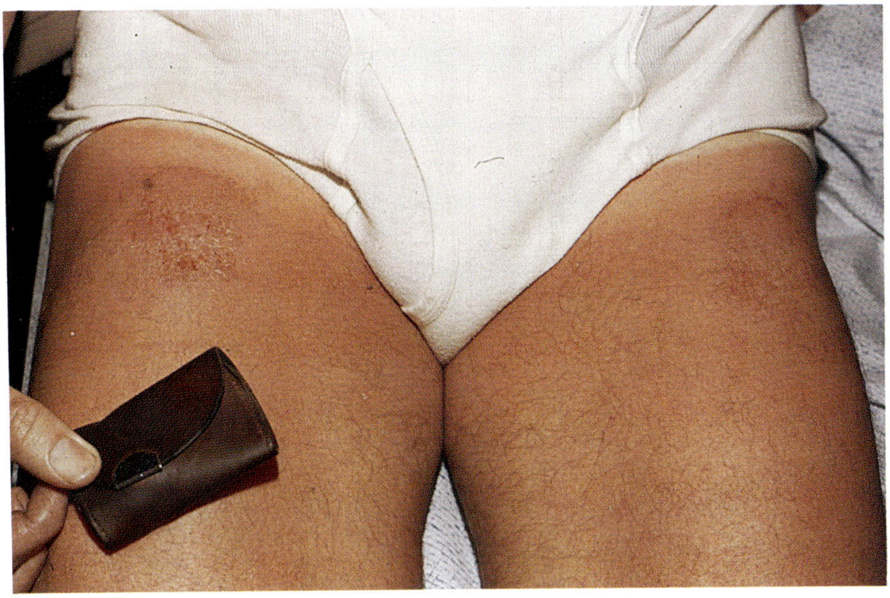

A

PARATERTIARY BUTYLPHENOL FORMALDEHYDE RESIN

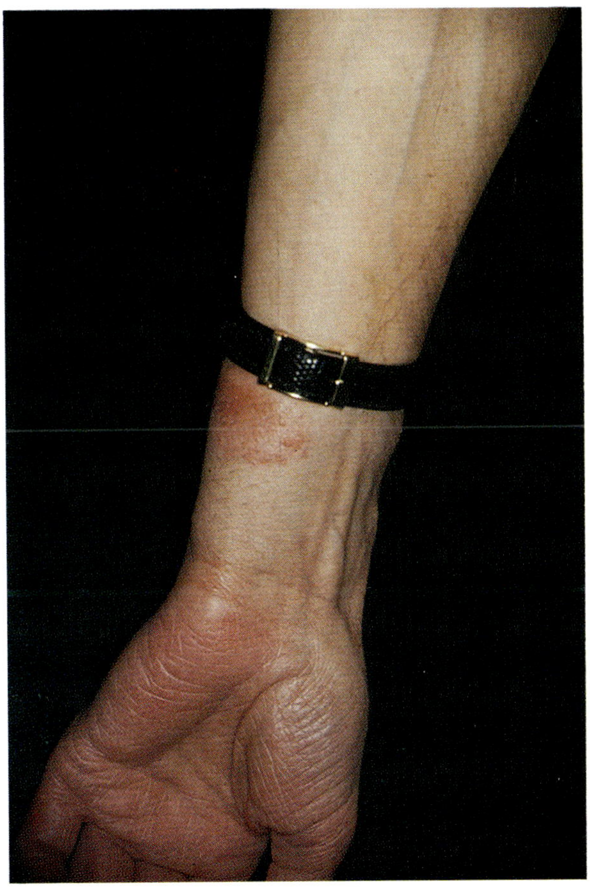

B

PARATERTIARY BUTYLPHENOL FORMALDEHYDE RESIN

COLOPHONY (ROSIN)

HISTORY

This middle-aged woman used a new eyeshadow and developed dermatitis several days later. Patch testing revealed a 2+ reaction to colophony.

RESOLUTION

Avoidance of colophony-containing cosmetics led to resolution of the dermatitis. Some months later, another dermatitis episode was traced to another eyeshadow. This points out the importance of carefully reading ingredient labeling on cosmetics and other preparations.

CLINICAL COMMENTS

The oxidation products of dehydroabietic acid are the principal sensitizers in colophony (rosin). Colophony is frequently found in adhesives, cosmetics, and medicaments. In industry, it is commonly found in soldering flux. It is a cause of dermatitis in workers in the semiconductor industry. Sensitivity to colophony has also been reported to affect string musicians using colophony (rosin) on their bows.

In this patient, sensitization had presumably occurred earlier, even though she could not recall a clinical episode.

References

Adams RM: Occupational Skin Disease, 2nd ed. Philadelphia, WB Saunders, 1990, p 421.
Fisher AA: Contact Dermatitis, 3rd ed. Philadelphia, Lea & Febiger, 1986, pp 424–426.
Hausen BM, Krohn K, Budianto E: Contact allergy due to colophony. VII. Sensitizing studies with oxidation products of abietic and related acids. Contact Dermatitis 23:352–358, 1990.
Karlberg AT, Bohlinder K, Boman A, et al: Identification of 15-hydroperoxyabietic acid as a contact allergen in Portuguese colophony. J Pharm Pharmacol 40:42–47, 1988.

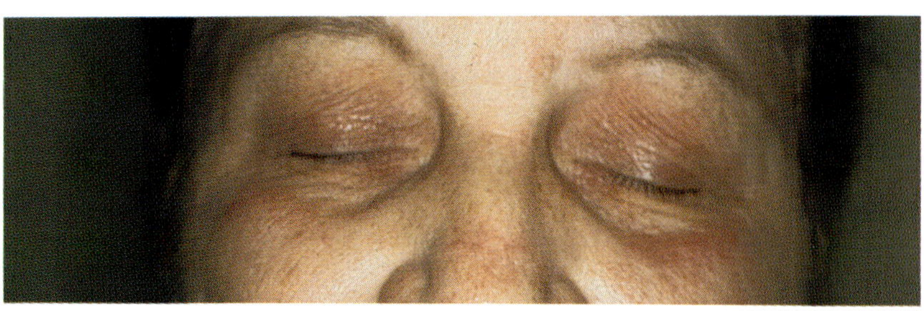

Courtesy of Alexander A. Fisher, M.D.

COLOPHONY (ROSIN)

Section II

Preservatives and Antibacterials

PARABENS

HISTORY

This patient had a leg ulcer treated with an Unna-type boot. The dermatitis gradually spread and became more severe. Eventually the dermatologist suspected the possibility of allergic contact dermatitis and patch tested the patient.

RESOLUTION

Patch testing revealed a positive reaction to the parabens mixture and to one component, propyl paraben. The leg ulcer continued to require therapy but the dermatitis noted here resolved with topical corticosteroid therapy and paraben avoidance.

CLINICAL COMMENTS

Presumably, paraben dermatitis was more common decades ago than today. It is possible that this was due to higher concentrations of paraben used in the past. This was certainly the case in countries such as Denmark, where the parabens used were in concentrations as high as 5% in topical agents. Fisher believes that patients testing positive to parabens who have a dermatitis such as leg ulcers may tolerate parabens on normal skin. Before recommending this, testing on an uninvolved skin area is indicated. Some cases of alleged paraben allergic contact dermatitis may have been reactions caused by the marginal irritancy of a mixture. For this reason, testing with the components is confirmatory.

Parabens are the most widely used preservatives for skin care products in the United States. Therefore, it is imperative that patients write down the names of the various parabens to which tests show they are sensitive.

Today paraben allergy is uncommon.

Reference

Fisher AA: Contact Dermatitis, 3rd ed. Philadelphia, Lea & Febiger, 1986, pp. 238–241.
Fisher AA: The paraben paradox. Cutis 12:830, 1973.

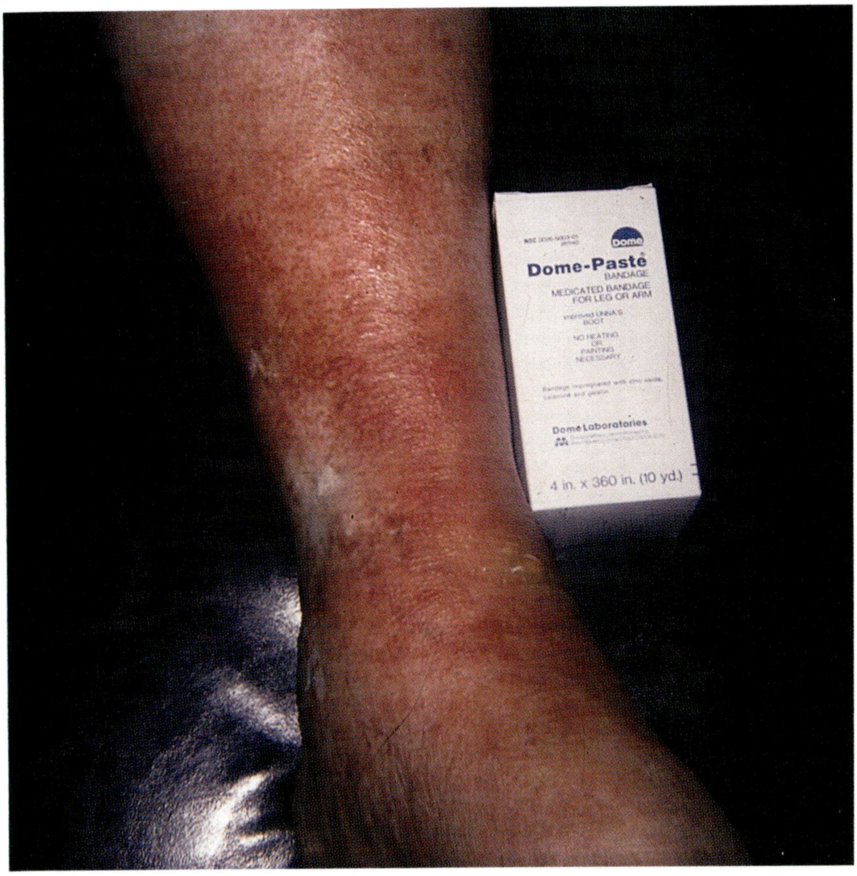

Courtesy of Frances J. Storrs, M.D.

PARABENS

2-BROMO-2-NITROPROPANE-1,3-DIOL (BRONOPOL)

HISTORY

This patient has a long-standing dermatitis that failed to respond to topical therapy. Because of its severity, a course of systemic prednisone was instituted. Because of the lesion morphology, the dermatologist patch tested the patient with the routine series, with preservatives, and with fragrances. The only relevant positive result was reaction to 2-bromo-2-nitropropane-1,3-diol (Bronopol).

RESOLUTION

After the diagnosis of allergic contact dermatitis from 2-bromo-2-nitropropane-1,3-diol (Bronopol, in Eucerin cream) was made, the patient promptly responded to corticosteroid therapy.

CLINICAL COMMENTS

The frequency of 2-bromo-2-nitropropane-1,3-diol (Bronopol) allergy is uncertain. Bronopol is not included in the routine testing series. At its usual patch test concentration it may be a marginal irritant. We do not know how much of this is due to lack of pharmaceutical homogeneity and how much to individual variation in irritancy response. For this reason, we perform a provocative use test with the preservative before stating to patients unequivocally that they are allergic. If the reaction is weak, we repeat the patch test before the provocative use test or repeat the open application test.

2-Bromo-2-nitropropane-1,3-diol is a formaldehyde releaser. Some patients are believed sensitive to it only; others to it and formalin.

Reference

Storrs FJ, Bell DE: Allergic contact dermatitis to 2-bromo-2-nitropropane-1,3 diol (Bronopol) in a hydrophilic ointment. J Am Acad Dermatol 8:157–170, 1983.

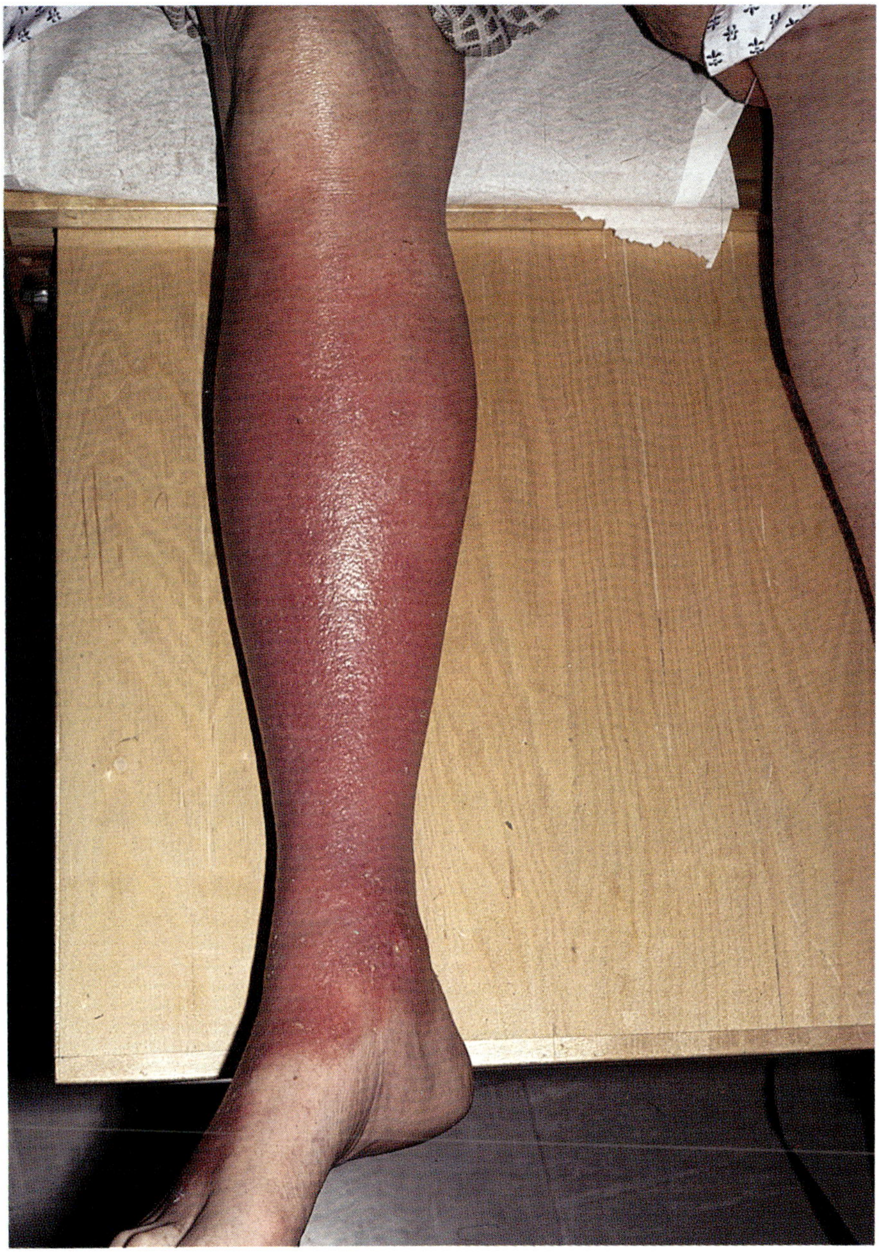

Courtesy of Frances J. Storrs, M.D.

2-BROMO-2-NITROPROPANE-1,3-DIOL (BRONOPOL)

ORTHO-PHENYLPHENOL

HISTORY

This 36-year-old man applied a popular body cream to his skin following bathing. He had used it previously for several weeks on his face and hands without difficulty. Within hours of the most recent application, he experienced severe, widespread itching, followed by a rash that in places was intense. Patch testing with the product "as is" and with its contents in nonirritant concentrations revealed a strong reaction to the product and to the preservative ortho-phenylphenol. Following treatment with systemic corticosteroids, the eruption rapidly cleared.

RESOLUTION

With ingredient labeling, the patient was able to avoid future contact with most substances containing ortho-phenylphenol. These include several common over-the-counter medications, germicidal agents present in cleaning agents for floors and walls, and certain cutting fluids used by machinists.

CLINICAL COMMENT

The dermatitis at first glance resembled poison oak or poison ivy dermatitis, but questioning revealed no possible contact with these plants. The manufacturer of the moisturizer was contacted and supplied each ingredient for testing, as well as samples of the product with and without ortho-phenylphenol.

References

Adams RM: Allergic contact dermatitis due to o-phenylphenol. Contact Dermatitis 7:332, 1981.
Cronin E: Contact Dermatitis. Edinburgh, Churchill Livingstone, 1980, p 681.

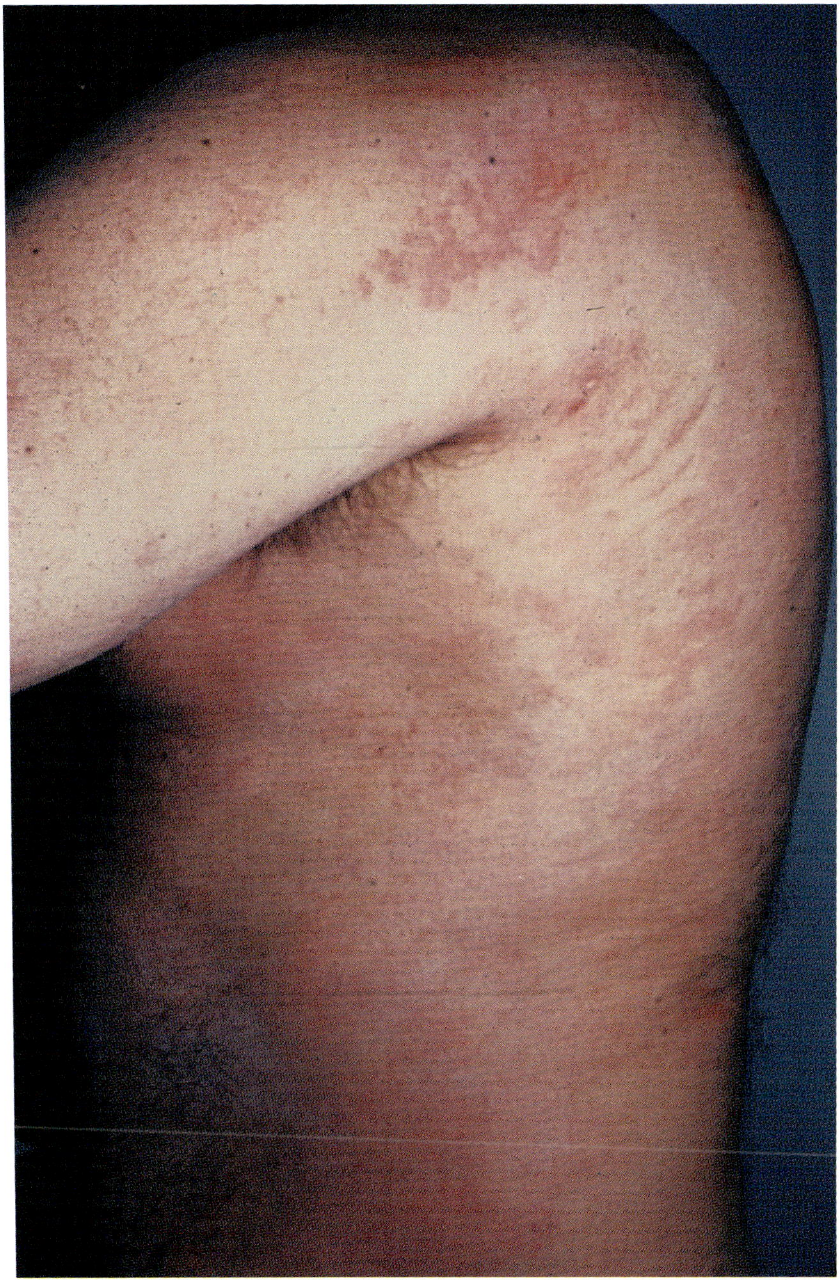

ORTHO-PHENYLPHENOL

GLUTARALDEHYDE

HISTORY

A 28-year-old respiratory technician developed a severely pruritic hand dermatitis. In his work, he handled the tubing and apparatus nearly equally with both hands. Patch testing revealed a strong positive reaction to glutaraldehyde, which was present in the germicidal agent Cidex that he used several times daily during his work cleaning and disinfecting the apparatus.

RESOLUTION

Glutaraldehyde is widely used as a cold sterilizer. Because the hospital refused to alter the cleaning methods and substitute a disinfectant without glutaraldehyde, the patient was compelled to change his occupation. His state's compensation system provided retraining.

CLINICAL COMMENT

This case illustrates the importance of establishing exact diagnosis through patch testing.

References

Adams RM: Occupational Skin Disease, 2nd ed. Philadelphia, WB Saunders, 1990, pp 629–630.
Goncalo S, Brandao FM, Pecegueiro M, et al: Occupational contact dermatitis to glutaraldehyde. Contact Dermatitis 10:183–184, 1984.
Hansen KS: Glutaraldehyde occupational dermatitis. Contact Dermatitis 9:81–82, 1983.
Jordan WP Jr, Dahl MV, Albert HL: Contact dermatitis from glutaraldehyde. Arch Dermatol 105:94–95, 1972.

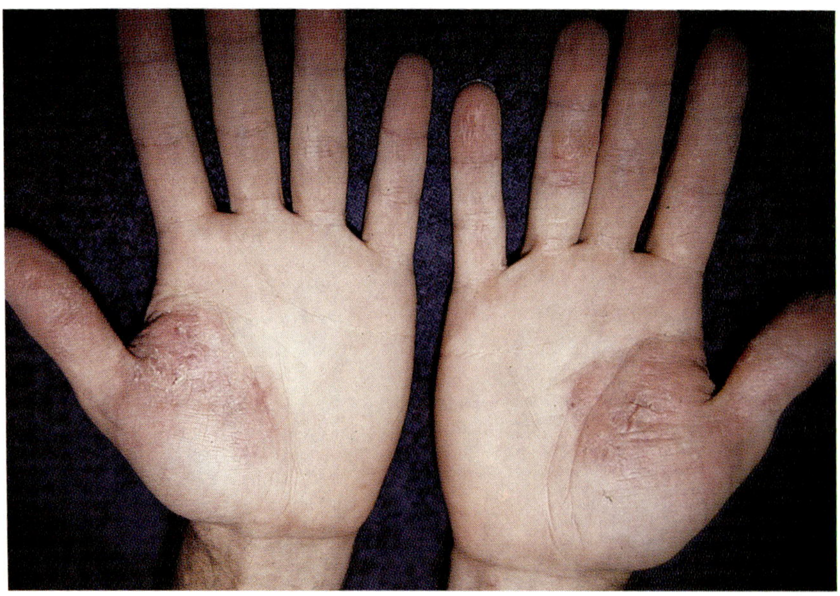

GLUTARALDEHYDE

Section III

Cosmetics and Skin Care Products

PRIMULA (*Primula obconica* Hance)

HISTORY

Every spring, this 45-year-old woman planted a row of primrose along her driveway. This year she selected a different variety, *Primula obconica*, which she found attractive. At first, after planting the flowers, which were already beginning to bloom, she noticed no rash. One month or so later, however, after pinching off dead leaves and blooms, she began to develop a red, weeping, intensely pruritic rash on the tips of her fingers, especially the thumb, index, and third fingers where she touched the leaves. Patch testing with both a small crushed piece of leaf and the allergenic chemical, primin (6-methoxy-2-N-pentyl-4-benzoquinone) at 0.01% in petrolatum, resulted in strong reactions.

RESOLUTION

The dermatitis responds rapidly to treatment with topical corticosteroids. The allergen, present in the fragile hairs on the ventral surface of the leaves, is potent and sensitivity long lasting. The only choice for sensitized primrose fanciers is to avoid *P. obconica* and its many varieties.

CLINICAL COMMENTS

The appearance of dermatitis on the tips of the first three fingers of the dominant hand in a person who is likely a gardener, and one who develops dermatitis during the 3- or 4-month growing season for primrose, means the person is a likely candidate. Other areas affected include the eyelids, neck, cheeks, arms, and so forth. The eruption may be highly pruritic and vesicular but often is of minimal intensity.

References

Benezra C, Ducombs G, Sell Y, et al: Plant Contact Dermatitis. St. Louis, CV Mosby, 1985, pp 200–201.

Hjorth N: Primula dermatitis: Sources of error in patch testing and patch test sensitization. Trans St Johns Hosp Dermatol Soc 52:207–219, 1966.

Rook A, Wilson HTH: Primula dermatitis. Br Med J i:220–222, 1965.

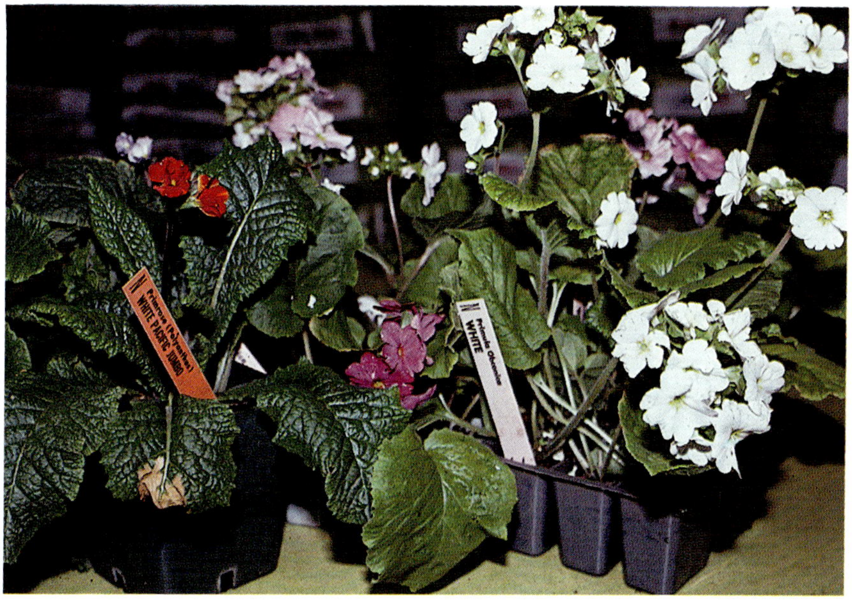

***PRIMULA OBCONICA* PLANT**

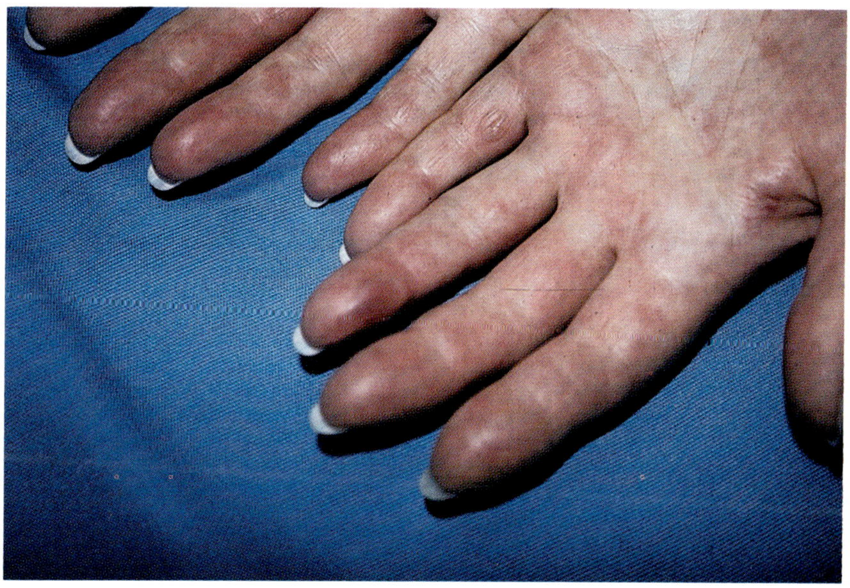

***PRIMULA OBCONICA* DERMATITIS**

RHUS (*TOXICODENDRON*): POISON IVY, POISON OAK, POISON SUMAC

These three pictures show the plant at different times of the year.

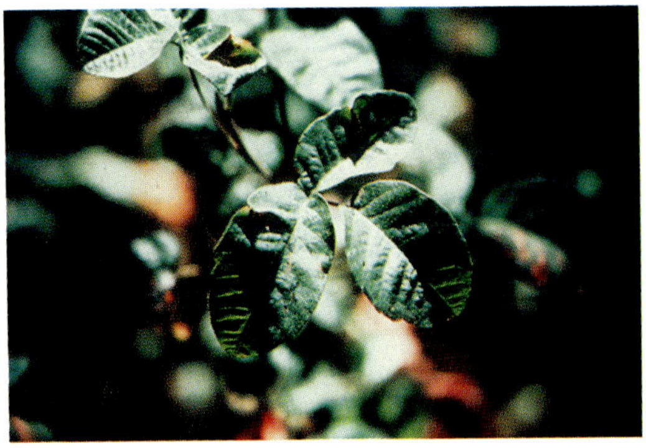

Courtesy of Frances J. Storrs, M.D.

RHUS *(TOXICODENDRON DIVERSILOBUM)*

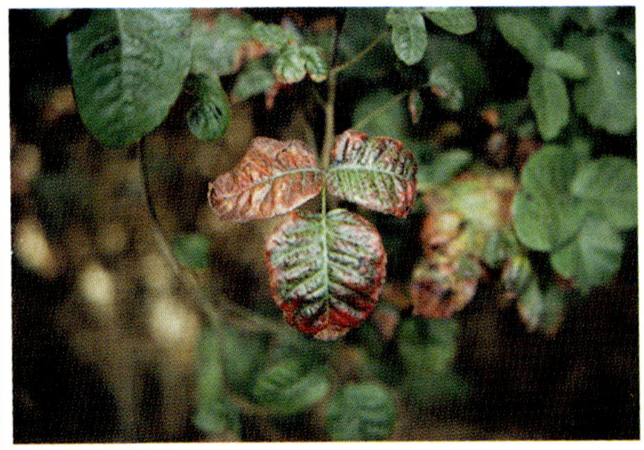

Courtesy of Frances J. Storrs, M.D.

RHUS IN AUGUST

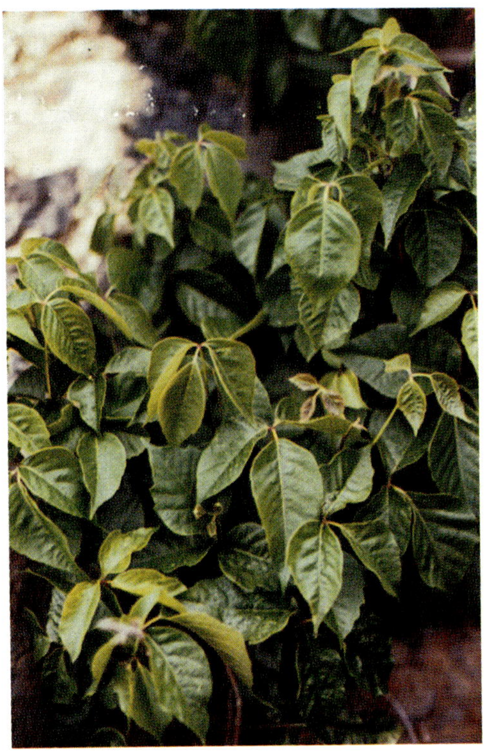

Courtesy of Frances J. Storrs, M.D.

RHUS VARIETY

HISTORY

Case I

This woman with no previous history of plant dermatitis had been working in her garden (*A*). These lesions developed several days later. The patient suspected plant dermatitis and sought emergency therapy.

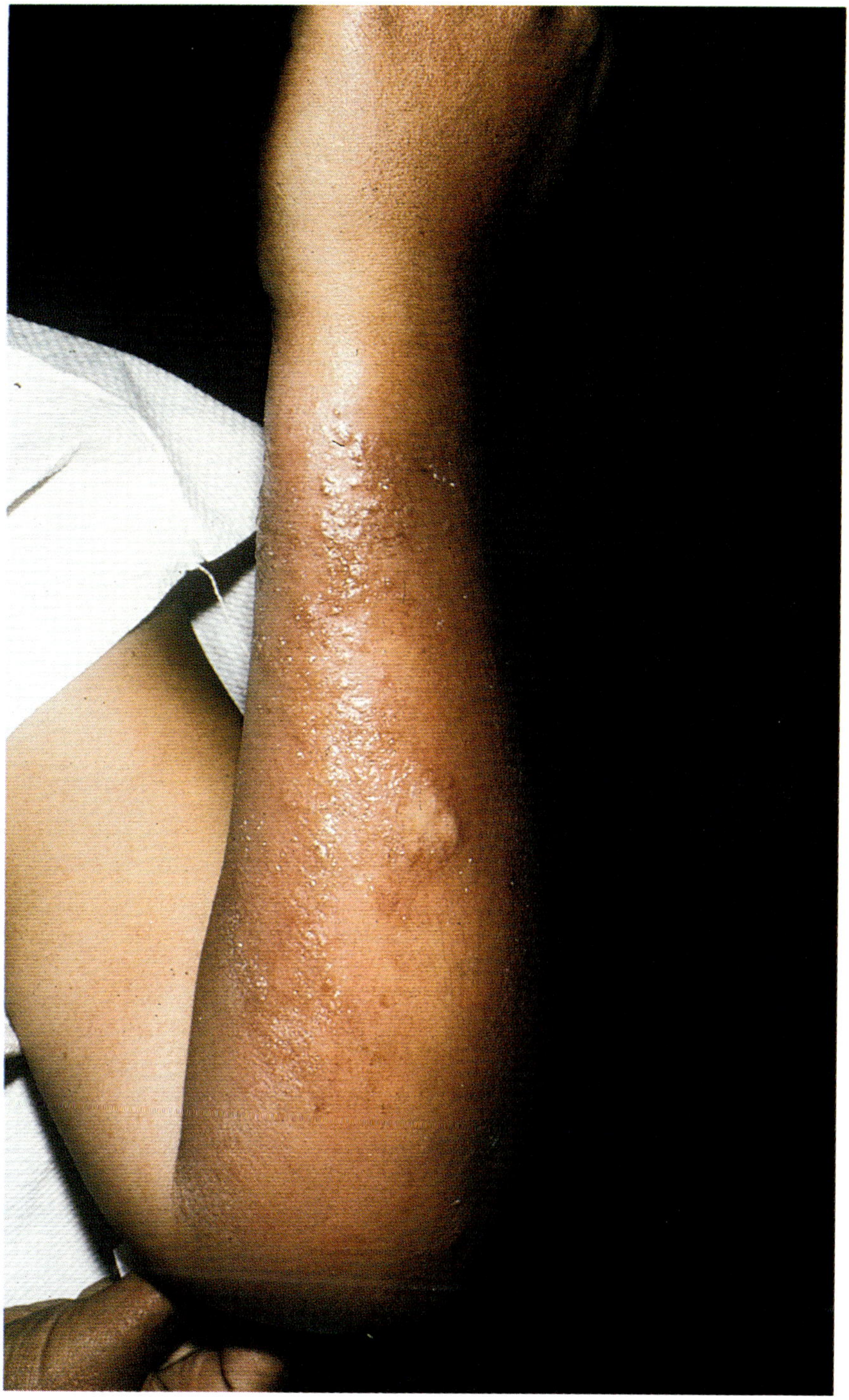

A

RHUS DERMATITIS

RHUS (*TOXICODENDRON*): POISON IVY, POISON OAK, POISON SUMAC *Continued*

Case II

These lesions developed on a camping trip in which there was presumably extensive exposure to poison oak on using outdoor toilet facilities (*B*).

Case III

This patient had been hiking in a short-sleeved shirt (*C*). The patient knew he was sensitive to Rhus but had not remembered touching the plant.

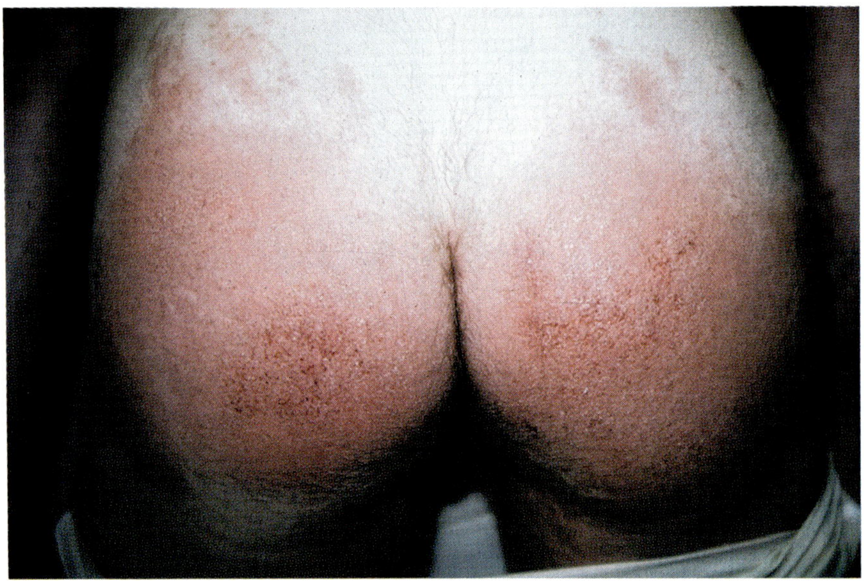

RHUS DERMATITIS

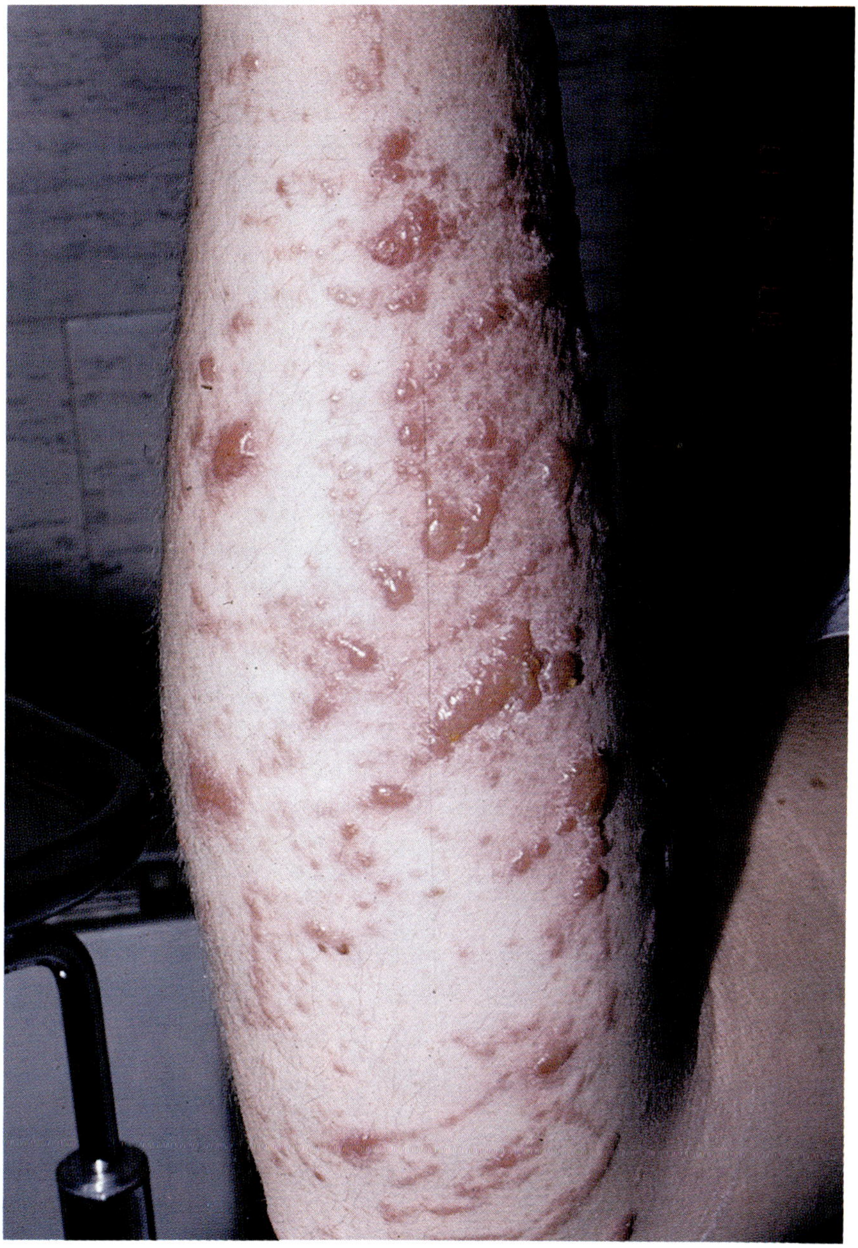

C

RHUS DERMATITIS

RHUS (*TOXICODENDRON*): POISON IVY, POISON OAK, POISON SUMAC *Continued*

Case IV

A recent arrival in Oregon, this woman did not know she was Rhus-sensitive. The present lesion developed 7 days after exposure (*D*).

These four photos demonstrate the varied morphology of poison oak dermatitis.

RESOLUTION

Rhus dermatitis clears spontaneously. Tap water compresses are generally effective. Topical corticosteroids, except in the late phases of the disease, or in mild disease, have only minimal efficacy. For patients who are disabled and extremely uncomfortable, systemic corticosteroids are almost immediately effective. Within 24 hours of systemic treatment most patients note marked symptomatic and early objective improvement. Prednisone in doses ranging from 40 to 80 mg is the typical treatment. If the drug is stopped early (that is, in 4 to 7 days) many patients have an exacerbation of symptoms.

CLINICAL COMMENTS

Rhus is the most common contact allergen in the United States and fortunately it is not present in Europe and many other countries, except in botanical gardens.

It is estimated that at least 50% of the United States population is sensitized in some states, such as California and Louisiana.

Once exposed, the patient will often, but not always, react to reexposure. On initial exposure, it may take 7 to 14 days or longer for lesions to be noted. It seems that many patients do not notice clinical symptoms on their sensitizing exposure.

Aiding the diagnosis are the linear dermatitic streaks; however, on the face, the edematous areas may be devoid of these streaks.

Many patients with Rhus dermatitis at first deny a history of exposure. This may be due to many factors, such as developing dermatitis from exposure to cat and dog fur containing bits of the resin.

Hyposensitization techniques are available and are effective when the patient is dosed to tolerance and continues hyposensitization. Unfortunately, within weeks of discontinuing the hyposensitization procedure, clinical sensitivity recurs.

The disease tends to become less severe and less common with increasing age. This is most noticeable in patients over 60 years of age.

References

Benezra C, Ducombs G, Sell Y, et al: Plant Contact Dermatitis. St Louis, CV Mosby, 1985.
Mitchell J, Rook A: Botanical Dermatology. Vancouver, Greengrass, 1979.

D
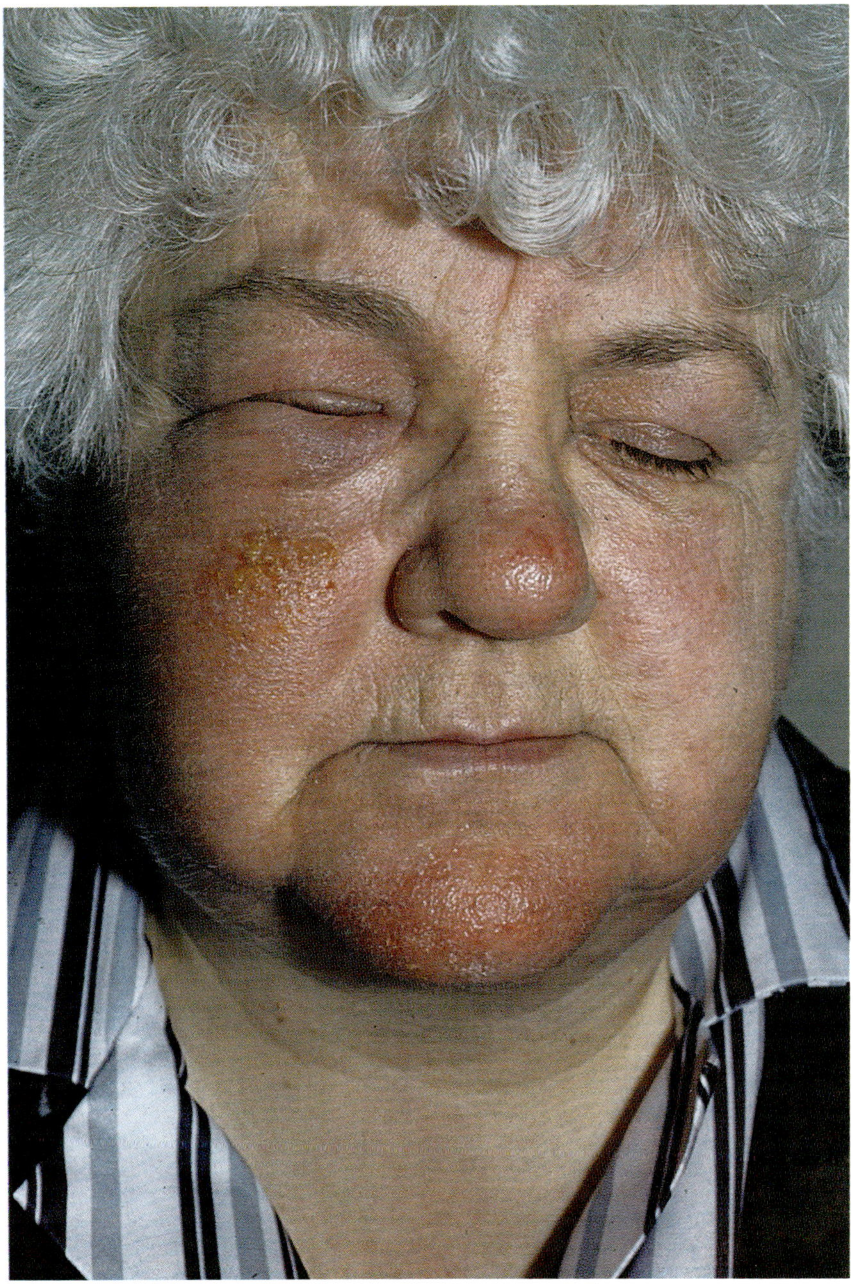

Courtesy of Frances J. Storrs, M.D.

RHUS DERMATITIS

Section V

Photodermatitis

MUSK AMBRETTE PERFUME

HISTORY

This man had a well demarcated bright red eruption on his face and neck. He had been using a well-known aftershave lotion for several months, but it was not until he was exposed to bright sunlight that the eruption suddenly developed.

RESOLUTION

Use of the aftershave lotion was discontinued and the patient was treated with topical and systemic corticosteroids. Clearing of the eruption required approximately 1 month. The manufacturer supplied the perfume, which on phototesting showed a strong positive reaction. Individual ingredients of the perfume were phototested, and ultimately it was determined that the offending photoallergen was musk ambrette.

CLINICAL COMMENTS

The first case of musk ambrette photoallergy was reported in 1978. Since that time, musk ambrette has been used in a screening photoallergen series, and many cases of musk ambrette photodermatitis have been detected. This photodermatitis tends to occur exclusively in men using aftershave lotion.

Musk ambrette is a synthetic chemical that has been used widely in cosmetics for the last 60 years. The International Fragrance Association has recommended that musk ambrette not be used in any cosmetic intended for use on the skin.

References

Raugi GH, Storrs FJ, Larsen WG: Photo allergic contact dermatitis to men's perfumes. Contact Dermatitis 5:251, 1979.

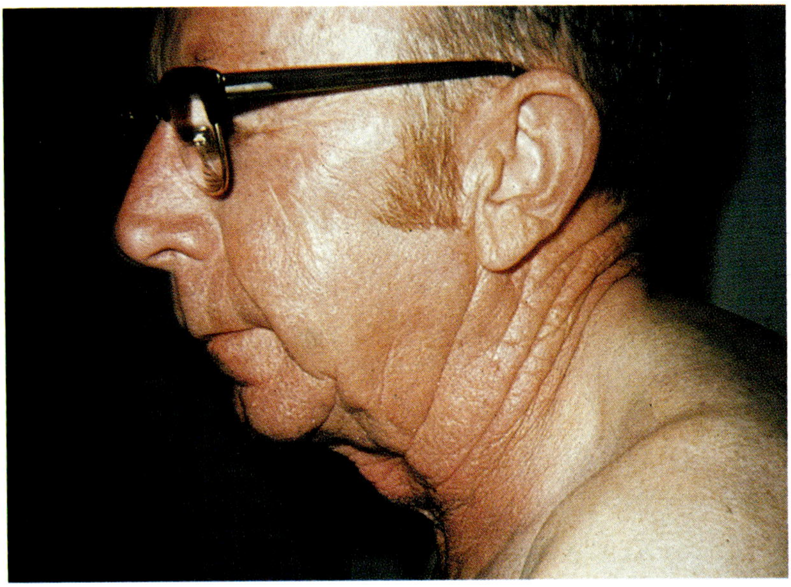

MUSK AMBRETTE PERFUME

OIL OF BERGAMOT

HISTORY

This young woman visited a suntan salon and the next day developed acute dermatitis on her neck and arms. The history revealed she had applied Shalimar perfume to the affected sites prior to ultraviolet (UV) exposure in the salon. The Shalimar perfume she used was 30 or 40 years old!

RESOLUTION

The acute eruption resolved very rapidly, but the pigmented areas remained for months. The Shalimar perfume, although very old, still contained the phototoxic ingredient oil of bergamot. The woman subsequently applied newly purchased Shalimar perfume and exposed herself to UV in the same suntan salon, but no reaction occurred.

CLINICAL COMMENTS

Approximately 20 years ago, phototoxic reactions to Shalimar and other perfumes containing oil of bergamot were common. However, almost all perfume manufacturers are now using bergapten-free oil of bergamot. The perfume industry is constantly trying to identify and eliminate other phototoxic photoallergens, such as rue oil, lemon oil, lime oil, and others.

Reference

Larsen WG: Perfume dermatitis. In Fisher AA: Contact Dermatitis, 3rd ed. Philadelphia, Lea & Febiger, 1986, pp 394–404.

Marzulli F, Maibach H: Photoirritation. In Marzulli F, Maibach H (eds.): Dermatotoxicology, 4th ed. Washington, DC, Hemisphere Press, 1991.

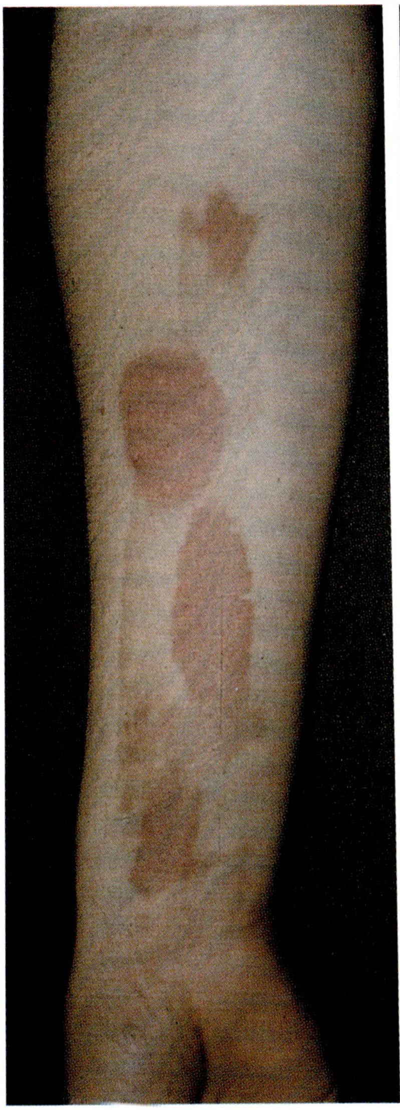

OIL OF BERGAMOT

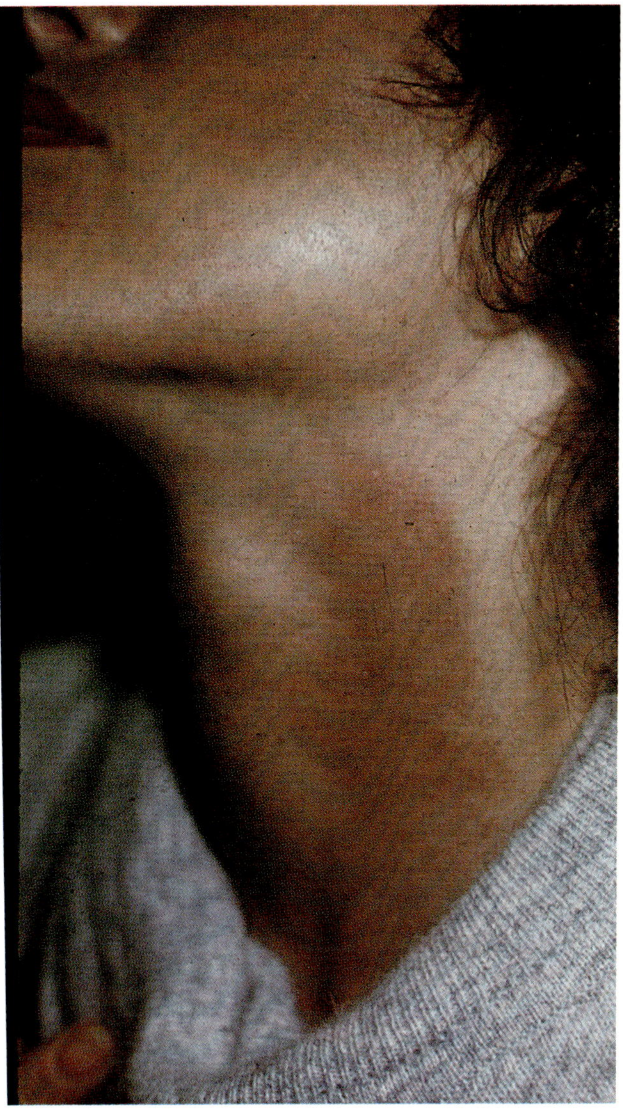

OIL OF BERGAMOT

BERLOQUE DERMATITIS

HISTORY

This woman applied perfume to her neck and chest and subsequently was exposed to sunlight. She developed an acute eruption that cleared with treatment, but hyperpigmentation persisted for many months.

RESOLUTION

This picture is typical of berloque dermatitis caused by certain perfumes, due to oil of bergamot, which contains bergapten, a psoralen. When perfume companies removed bergapten, the incidence of this dermatitis in consumers virtually disappeared. The hallmark of this reaction is hyperpigmentation, which persists for a long time.

CLINICAL COMMENTS

Many natural products cause this type of reaction when applied to the skin that is then exposed to sunlight. These products include celery, lime, lemon, parsnip, and rue. Each contains psoralen, which is a potent phototoxic agent. Perfume manufacturers have attempted to eliminate all psoralen-containing materials from their products.

Reference

Harber LC, et al: Berloque dermatitis. Arch Dermatol 90:572, 1964.

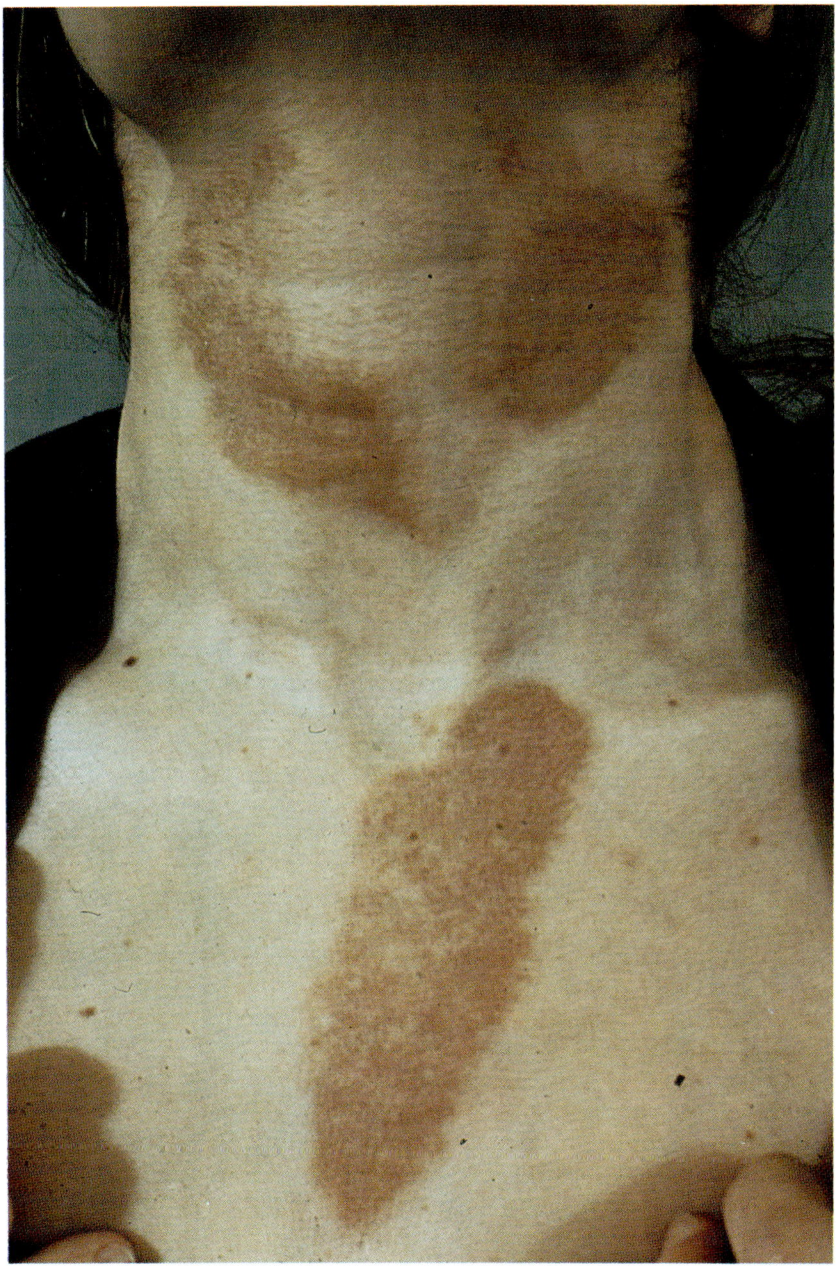

Courtesy of Donald V. Belsito, M.D.

BERLOQUE DERMATITIS

PHOTOIRRITATION (PHOTOTOXICITY)

HISTORY

Case I

This patient had been preparing mixed drinks outdoors near the noon hour (*A*). Contact included alcohol, soft drinks, and limes.

Case II

This patient had been handling celery in a grocery store and had been exposed to late afternoon sun (*B*).

RESOLUTION

Both cases were believed, on the basis of history and morphology, to be due to photoirritation. Both cleared with tap water compresses and use of a topical corticoid agent. Postinflammatory hyperpigmentation lasted many months.

CLINICAL COMMENTS

The mechanism of photoirritation was clarified in the late 1960s when it was realized that ultraviolet A (UVA) was the eliciting factor in almost all cases.

The second advance in understanding classical bergamot hypersensitivity was that it was sometimes necessary not only to use UVA but to apply the chemical to damaged skin. Cellophane tape stripping is the standard method to increase sensitivity. The amount of time between exposure to the chemical and exposure to the UVA is variable.

In practice, it is uncommon to test for photoirritation in an office setting. Most studies are done using preclinical toxicologic assays and knowledge of the wavelengths of the material or its metabolites.

Phototoxicity may be insidious. For years amyldimethyl paraamino benzoic acid (PABA) was utilized as a sunscreen before it was understood that it is a photoirritant.

Until there is more complete screening for irritation, we will continue to be surprised about materials that are photoirritants.

References

Marzulli F, Maibach H: Dermatotoxicology, 4th ed. Washington, DC, Hemisphere Press, 1991.

A

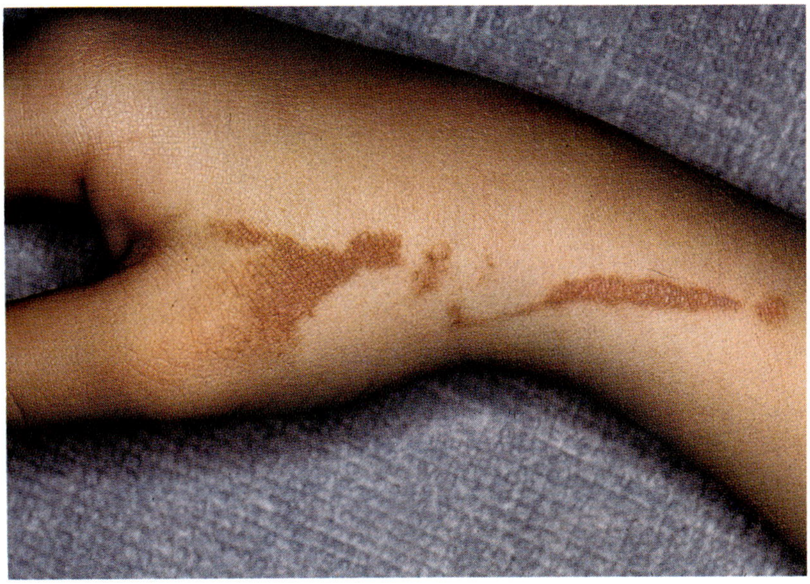

Courtesy of Alexander A. Fisher, M.D.

PHOTOIRRITATION (PHOTOTOXICITY)

B

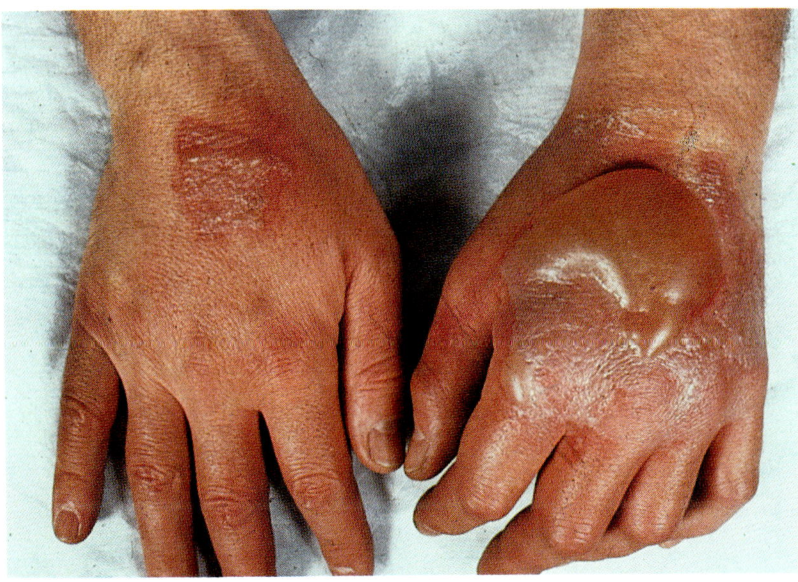

Courtesy of Donald V. Belsito, M.D.

PHOTOIRRITATION (PHOTOTOXICITY)

LIME

HISTORY

A 15-year-old girl spent a sunny afternoon at the beach, squeezing limes to make limeade for her friends. Within several hours she noticed burning and stinging on the dorsam of her hands and wrists, and by the next morning there was blistering. Within a few weeks a blotchy hyperpigmentation appeared on the affected areas.

RESOLUTION

Following a few days of treatment and avoidance of further sunlight, the acute reaction subsided. Hyperpigmentation required several months to disappear.

CLINICAL COMMENTS

The rind of lime contains bergamot oil, which contains a psoralen, 5-methoxy psoralen (5-MOP), capable of inducing a phytophotodermatitis when exposed to sunlight. The reaction is phototoxic rather than photoallergic. A burning sensation is often a more prominent symptom than is pruritus, and the reaction varies directly with the amount of sunlight exposure. The action spectrum is UVA.

References

Emmett EA: Phototoxicity and photosensitivity reactions. In Adams RM (ed.): Occupational Skin Disease, 2nd ed. Philadelphia, WB Saunders, 1990, p 185.

Marzulli F, Maibach H: Phototoxicity. In Marzulli F, Maibach M: Dermatotoxicology, 4th ed. Washington, DC, Hemisphere Press, 1991.

Sams WM: Photodynamic action of lime oil *(C. aurantifolia)*. Arch Dermatol Syph 44:571–587, 1941.

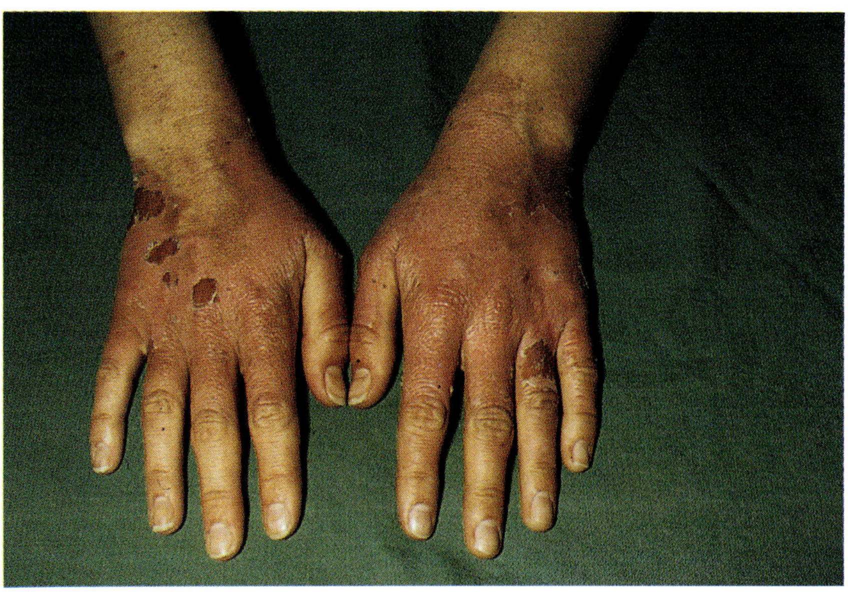

LIME

Section VI

Clothing and Textiles

CLOTHING

HISTORY

This 38-year-old businessman developed a pruritic dermatitis on his trunk, arms, and legs following purchase of a new, expensive suit of clothes. The dermatitis cleared to some extent on weekends but recurred a day or two following return to work. Patch testing to standard allergens revealed a strong positive reaction to formaldehyde, 1% aqueous, and further testing showed positive reactions to urea formaldehyde resin (10% in petrolatum) and to dimethyloldihydroxyethylene urea (10% in petrolatum).

RESOLUTION

The dermatitis continued for several months but gradually disappeared following several dry cleanings of his suits. He regularly had dry cleaned any new suits purchased, and all new clothing (and bedsheets) were washed several times prior to use.

CLINICAL COMMENTS

Clothing dermatitis due to formaldehyde finishes decreased in frequency during the 1980s, but recently it has shown an increase, probably because more fabric is manufactured overseas by companies unaware of the importance of removing residues of the resins prior to shipment to clothing manufacturers. The dermatitis tends to be rather dry, scaling, erythematous, and prominent in areas of pressure, such as the axillary areas (sparing the vault), the flanks, and inner thighs.

Fabrics such as 100% cotton denim, 100% silk, 100% linen (the type that wrinkles), 100% wool, 100% polyester, 100% nylon, and 100% ultrasuede are unlikely to be finished with formaldehyde resins.

References

Cronin E: Clothing and textiles. In Cronin E: Contact Dermatitis. Edinburgh, Churchill Livingstone, 1980, pp 36–92.

Fowler JF Jr, Skinner SM, Belsito DV: Allergic contact dermatitis from resins in permanent press clothing: An underdiagnosed cause of generalized dermatitis. In press.

Storrs FJ: Dermatitis from clothing and shoes. In Fisher AA: Contact Dermatitis, 3rd ed. Philadelphia, Lea & Febiger, 1986, pp 283–337.

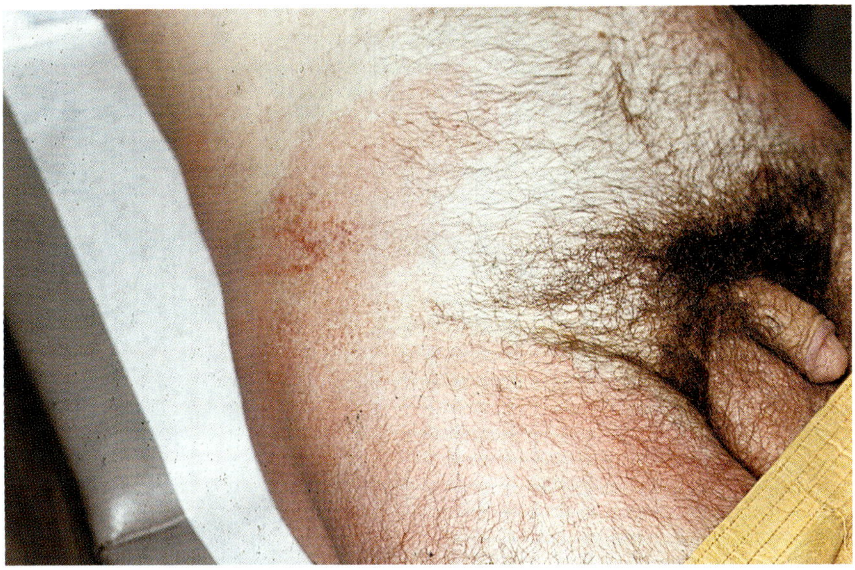

NEW CLOTHING

DISPERSE DYES

HISTORY

A pruritic dermatitis developed in this middle-aged woman when she wore a new pair of stockings. The eruption was severe and persisted for several weeks even with extensive treatment consisting of topical and systemic corticosteroids. Patch testing to numerous clothing allergens revealed strong positive reactions to disperse blue 3 and 7, and disperse yellow 3, each at 1% concentration in petrolatum.

RESOLUTION

Wearing 100% cotton socks is a safe substitution.

CLINICAL COMMENTS

The numerous disperse dyes are the chief cause of allergic contact dermatitis from clothing. The dermatitis is usually very pruritic, but often shows little vesiculation. Diagnosis may be suggested by the characteristic pattern under the clothing.

References

Cronin E: Studies in contact dermatitis. XIX: Nylon stocking dyes. Trans St Johns Hosp Dermatol Soc 54:165, 1968.

Hatch K, Maibach H: Textile fiber dermatitis. Contact Dermatitis 12:1–11, 1985.

Storrs F: Dermatitis from clothing and shoes. In Fisher AA (ed): Contact Dermatitis, 3rd ed. Philadelphia, Lea & Febiger, 1986, pp 306–313.

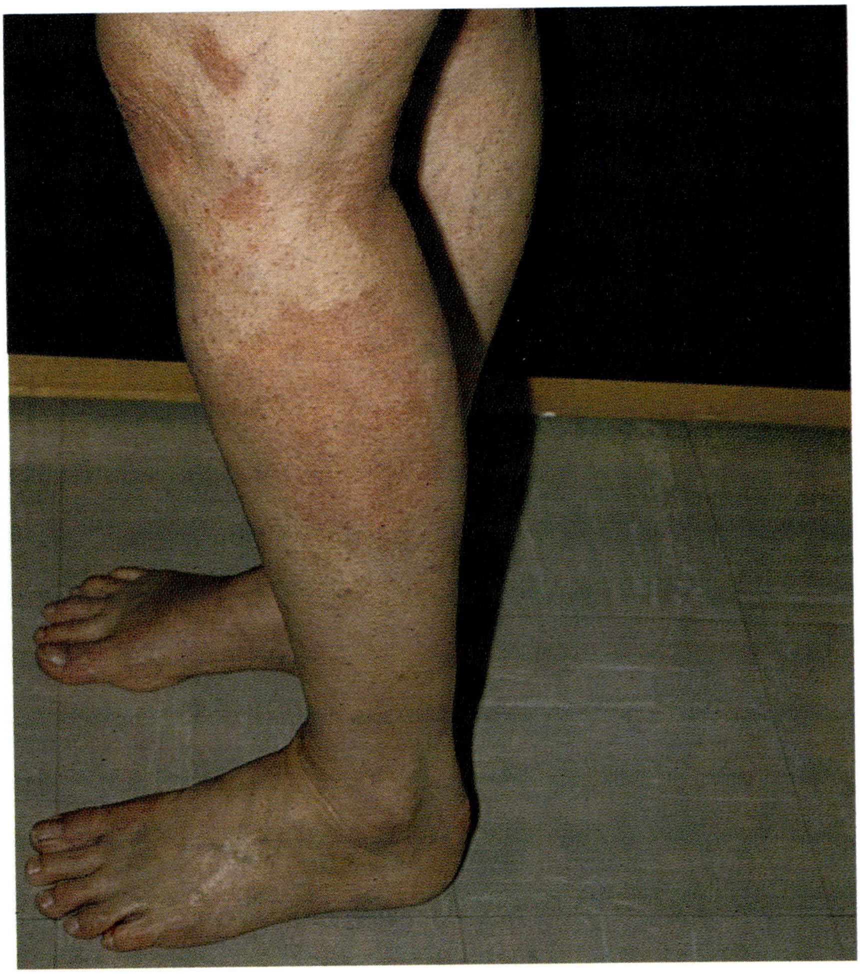

Courtesy of Frances J. Storrs, M.D.

DISPERSE DYE IN STOCKINGS

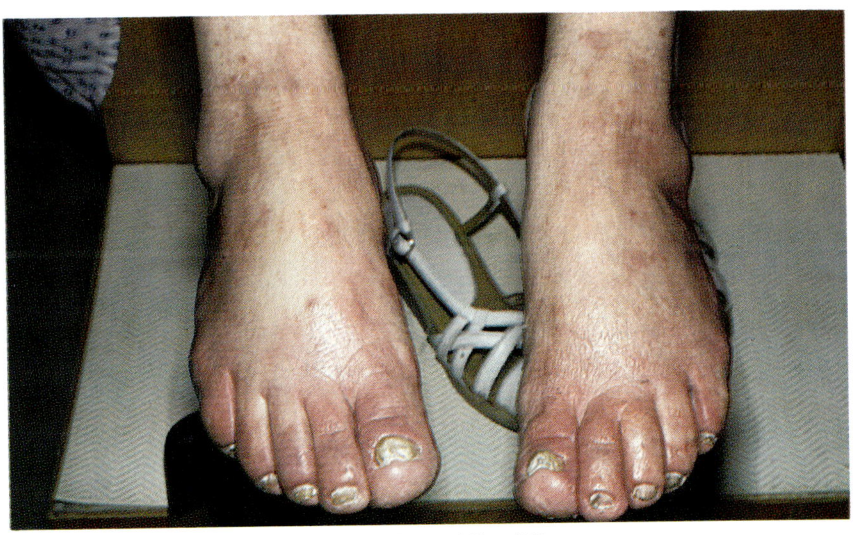

Courtesy of Frances J. Storrs, M.D.

DISPERSE DYE IN STOCKINGS

TEXTILE DERMATITIS

HISTORY

A 41-year-old female physician had a 4-month history of pruritic axillary eruption, sparing the vault, that was unresponsive to topical corticosteroid treatment. Patch testing revealed strong reactions to a flannel nightgown and a polyester jumper, and also to formaldehyde, Quaternium-15, ethylene urea/melamine formaldehyde, dimethyloldihydroxyethylene urea, dimethylolpropylene urea, tetramethylolacetylene diurea, and ethylene urea.

RESOLUTION

Multiple washings and dry cleaning usually reduce the level of these formaldehyde-based resins. The wearing of 100% cotton garments, or 100% polyester "non-drip dry" clothing, is also helpful. Weight reduction and control of hyperhidrosis are also important therapeutic measures.

CLINICAL COMMENTS

Clothing dermatitis characteristically involves areas of skin in greatest contact with the fabric. The vault of the axilla is nearly always spared. The rash is usually pruritic but not markedly vesicular. Patch testing with formaldehyde is usually positive, and the diagnosis can be confirmed by testing with the above clothing finishes.

Reference

Storrs F: Dermatitis from clothing and shoes. In Fisher AA (ed): Contact Dermatitis, 3rd ed. Philadelphia, Lea & Febiger, 1986, pp 283–337.

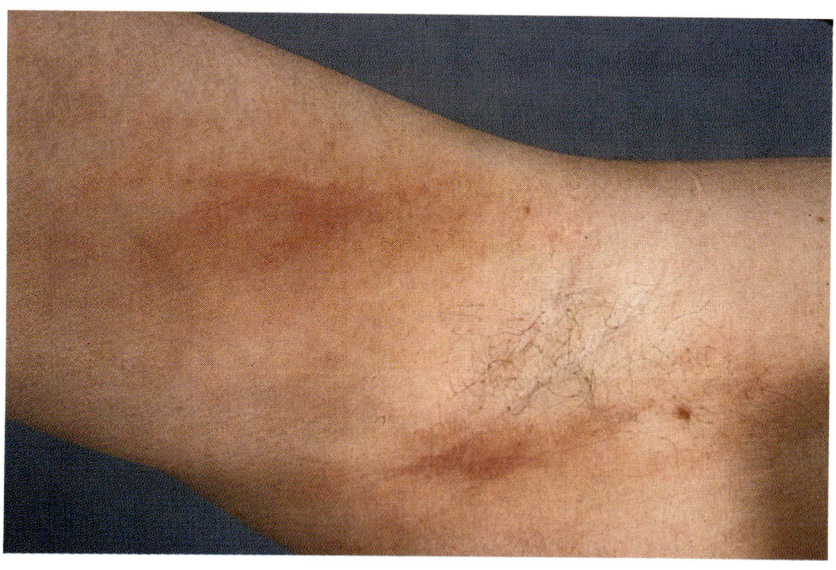

Courtesy of Donald V. Belsito, M.D.

TEXTILE DERMATITIS

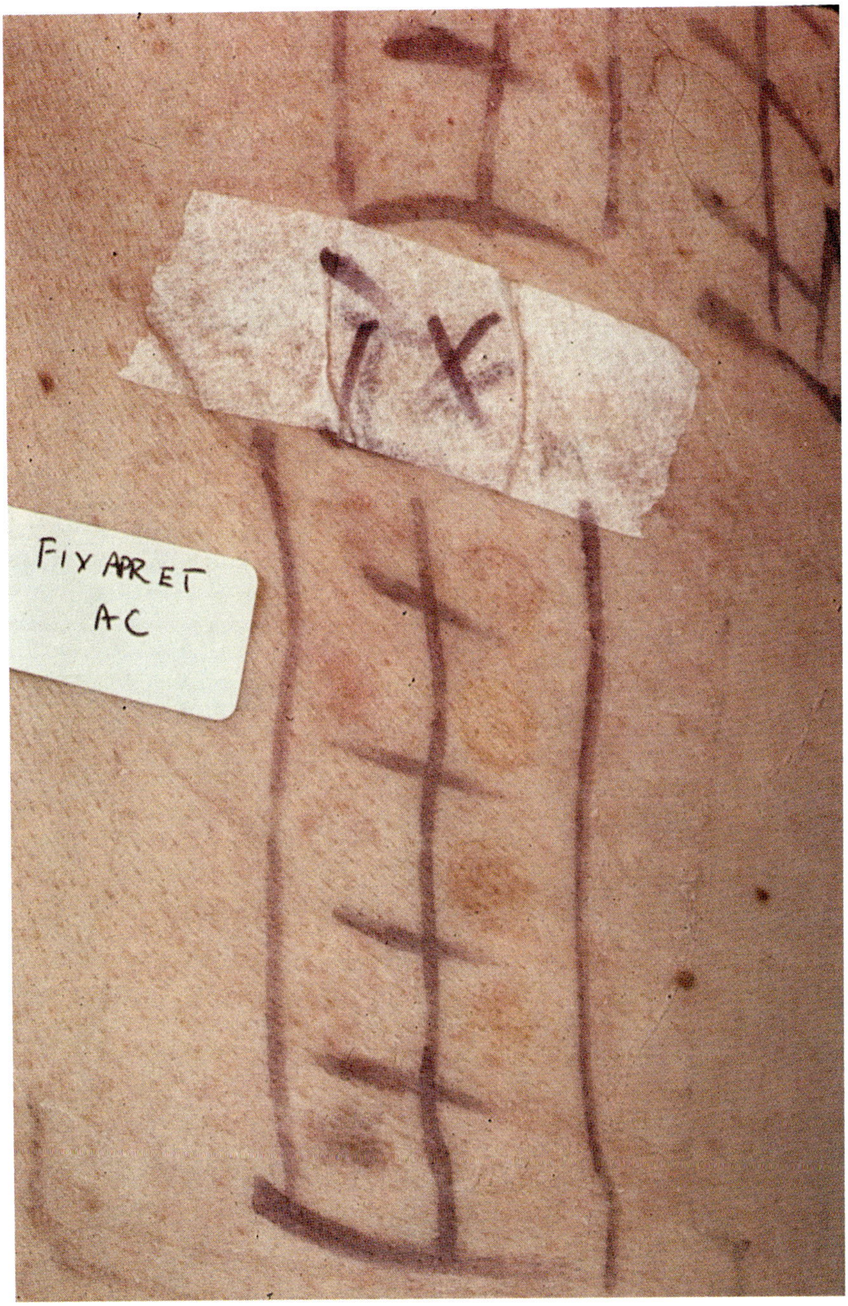

PATCH TESTING REACTIONS TO TEXTILE RESINS

Section VII

Rubber Chemicals

STETHOSCOPE

HISTORY

This nurse had recurrent dermatitis on the back of her neck. Routine series patch testing revealed a positive reaction to mercaptobenzothiazole.

RESOLUTION

The lesions cleared on having the nurse switch to using plastic tubing.

RESPIRATORY MASK

HISTORY

A 43-year-old auto mechanic developed dermatitis of the dorsa of both hands several years ago. A diagnosis of allergic contact dermatitis was made and patch testing revealed a strongly positive reaction to mercaptobenzothiazole (1% in petrolatum), which was presumed present in the rubber gloves he wore intermittently. He changed his type of work and began employment in the semiconductor industry. He did well for a time but developed dermatitis on the face after beginning to wear a respirator with a rubber face mask. Patch testing to a piece of the face mask and a repeat test with mercaptobenzothiazole were positive.

RESOLUTION

This was an easy solution. The worker merely changed to a face mask made of silicone "rubber," which does not contain the usual rubber allergens including mercaptobenzothiazole, and his dermatitis cleared and remained clear.

CLINICAL COMMENTS

Mercaptobenzothiazole is still a common rubber allergen, although sensitivity has become less frequent in recent years. At one time it was the most common allergen in shoes and may still be seen occasionally, especially in the inner soles of imported shoes. It should be considered in almost all contact allergic dermatitis where rubber is in contact with the skin.

References

Brandao FM: Rubber. In Adams RM (ed): Occupational Skin Disease, 2nd ed. Philadelphia, WB Saunders, 1990, pp 462–485.

Guin J: The MBT paradox. Am J Contact Dermatitis, Sept, 1990, pp 195–197.

Taylor JS: Rubber. In Fisher AA: Contact Dermatitis, 3rd ed. Philadelphia, Lea & Febiger, 1986, pp 603–643.

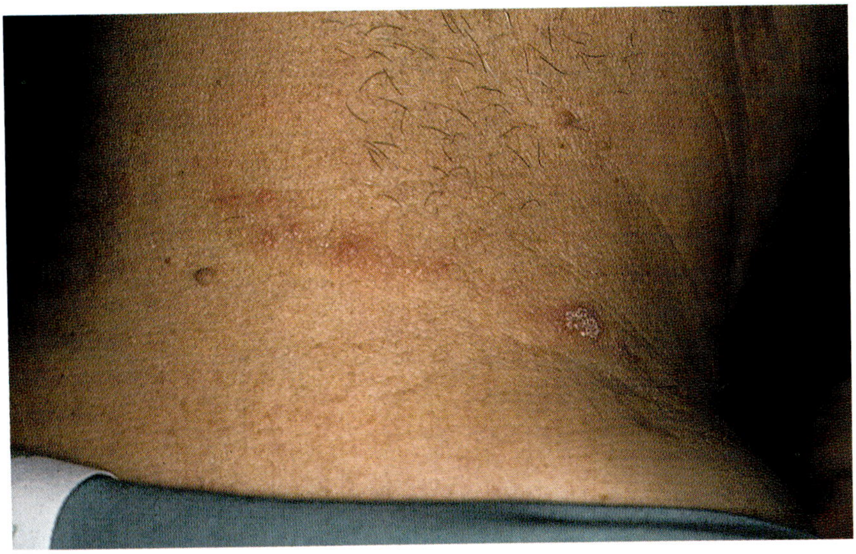

Courtesy of Robert L. Rietschel, M.D.

STETHOSCOPE

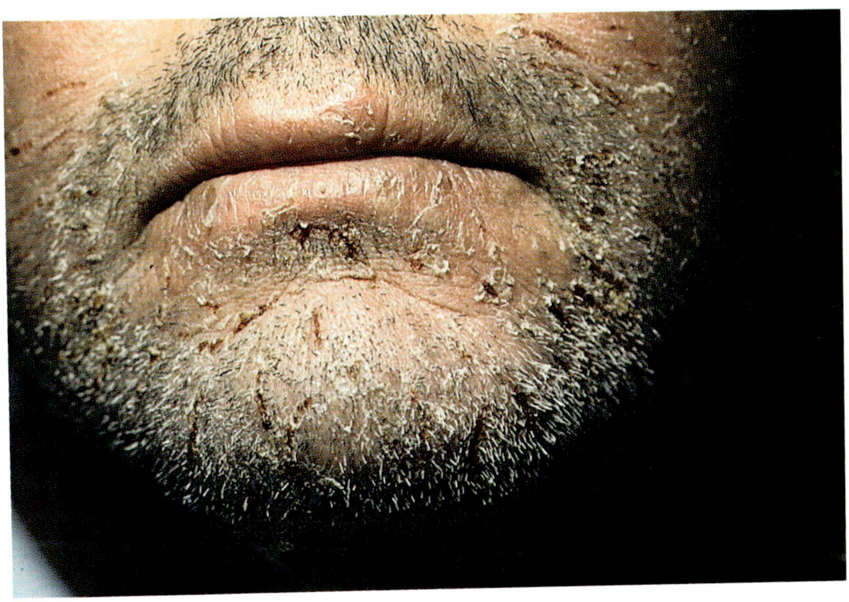

RESPIRATORY MASK

WET SUIT

HISTORY

After working as a professional diver for several years, this 28-year-old man developed a severe, widespread, pruritic dermatitis under his rubber wet suit. Patch testing to a small piece of the suit was positive. Testing with allergens on the standard tray was negative, but patch testing to diethyl and dibutyl thioureas, 1% in petrolatum, revealed strongly positive reactions.

RESOLUTION

The manufacturer of the wet suit stated that these thioureas were used in the manufacture of the suit's rubber and suggested the patient confine his wearing to another suit not containing these rubber accelerators. With this knowledge, the diver instructed his company to purchase only the recommended suit. As a result, he continued work without further dermatitis. On one occasion, however, after wearing another suit borrowed from a colleague for only a few hours, a severe dermatitis required that he be hospitalized.

CLINICAL COMMENTS

The thioureas are used primarily for soft, sponge-type rubber used in clothing, orthopedic appliances, sometimes in inner soles of shoes, and in rubber insulation for pipe, roofing, and other industrial uses. They are potent allergens that produce a markedly inflammatory dermatitis.

References

Adams RM: Contact allergic dermatitis due to diethylthiourea in a wet suit. Contact Dermatitis 8:277–279, 1982.

Brandao FM: Rubber. In Adams, RM (ed): Occupational Skin Disease, 2nd ed. Philadelphia, WB Saunders, 1990, pp 462–485.

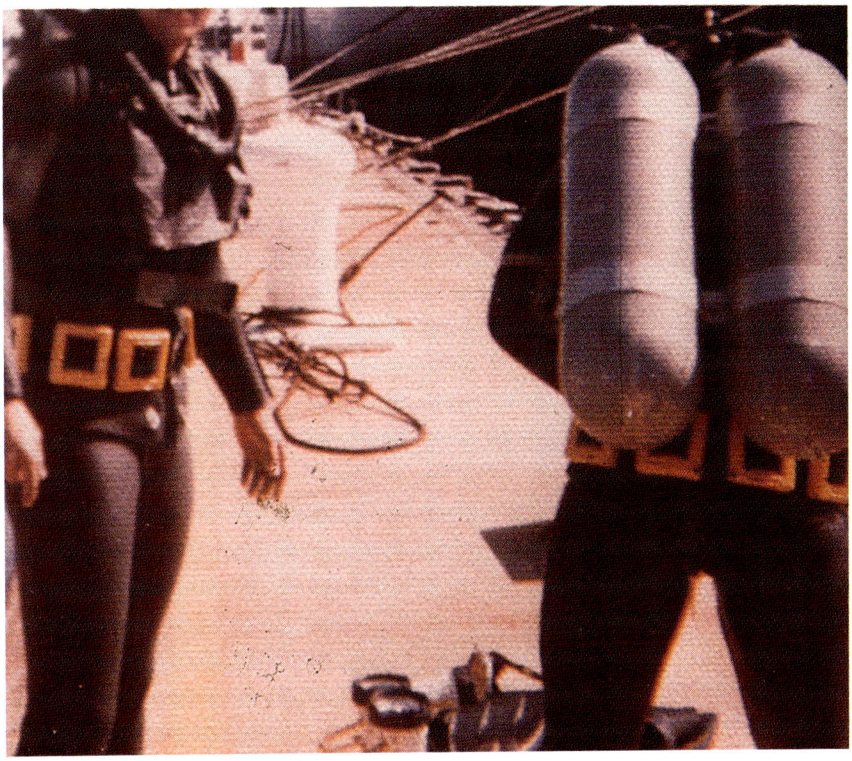

WET SUIT

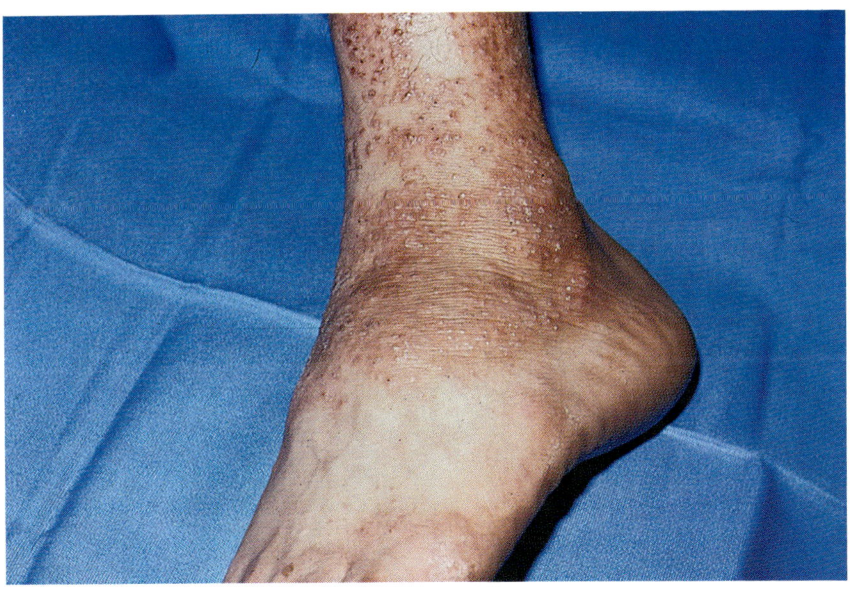

WET SUIT

ELASTIC BAND

HISTORY

This man had an eruption around his waist. The outline of the eruption completely fit that of the elastic waistband of his shorts. Patch testing revealed a positive reaction to the rubber in the elastic band of the shorts. A patch test of a research material (N-N-dibenzyl carbamyl chloride) was positive. His wife had recently begun to use bleach in the laundry.

RESOLUTION

The patient was advised not to use bleach when washing the shorts.

CLINICAL COMMENTS

The rubber in the unbleached shorts was not allergenic. Bleaching produced a new rubber chemical that was allergenic (N-N-dibenzyl carbamyl chloride).

Reference

Jordan WP Jr, Bourlas MC: Allergic Contact dermatitis to underwear elastic. Arch Dermatol 111:593, 1975.

SPANDEX RUBBER BRASSIERE

HISTORY

This woman had developed an insidious dermatitis that previously had been diagnosed as nonspecific eczema and tinea. Patch testing to the routine test series revealed a positive reaction to mercaptobenzothiazole. Testing to the garment itself, containing the synthetic material spandex, was positive.

RESOLUTION

The dermatitis cleared rapidly when a non-mercaptobenzothiazole-containing brassiere was substituted.

CLINICAL COMMENTS

Mercaptobenzothiazole is no longer used in spandex. Thus it can now be safely used as a rubber substitute for patients sensitive to rubber additives. Spandex is lighter and whiter than rubber and thus has advantages for swim suits and underwear.

Reference

Porter PS, Sommer RG: Contact dermatitis due to Spandex. Arch Dermatol 95:43, 1967.

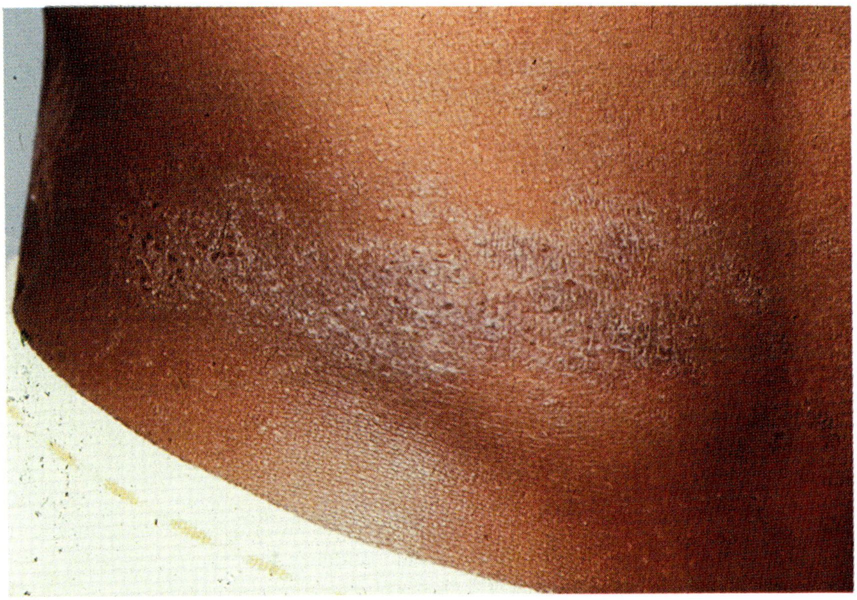

Courtesy of William P. Jordan, M.D.

ELASTIC BAND

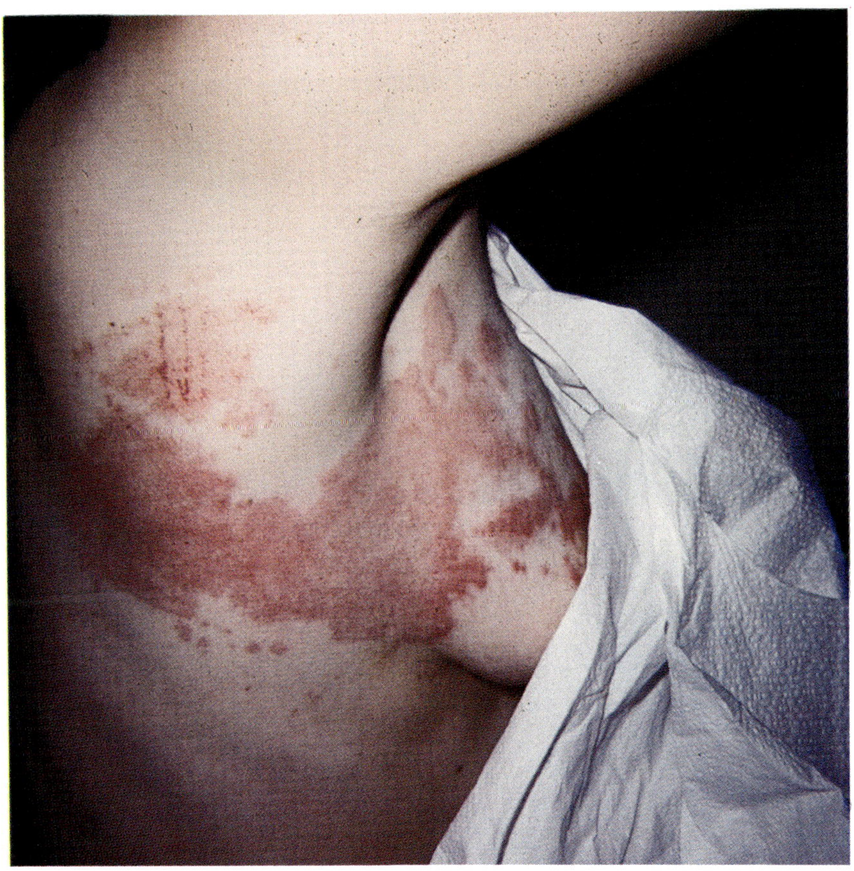

SPANDEX RUBBER BRASSIERE

SHOES

HISTORY

Case I

This patient had chronic eruption of the soles, diagnosed variously as tinea and nonspecific eczema (*A*). A patch test with the patient's shoe insert was positive.

Case II

This patient had chronic dermatitis of the sole (*B*). This was variously diagnosed as tinea and nonspecific eczema. A patch test was positive with the top of the sandals shown.

Case III

This patient had chronic dermatitis treated for many months as chronic eczema (*C*). Patch testing was positive with the top of the shoe shown and with individual rubber chemicals.

A

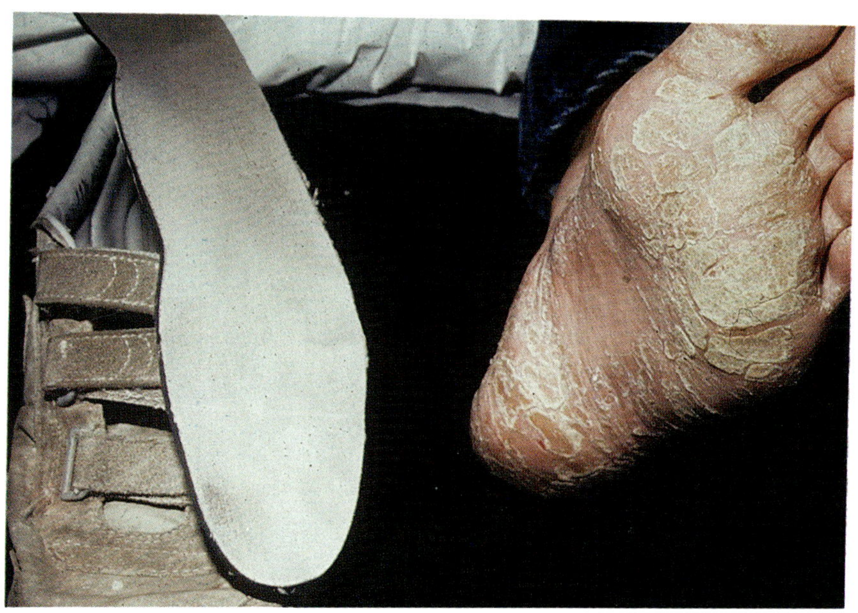

Courtesy of Frances J. Storrs, M.D.

SHOE INSERT

B
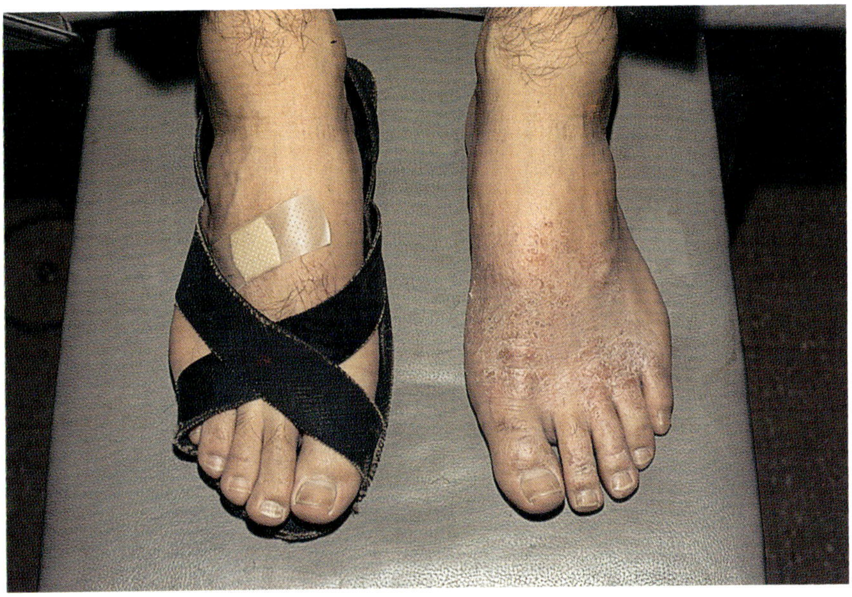

Courtesy of Frances J. Storrs, M.D.

SHOE TOP

C
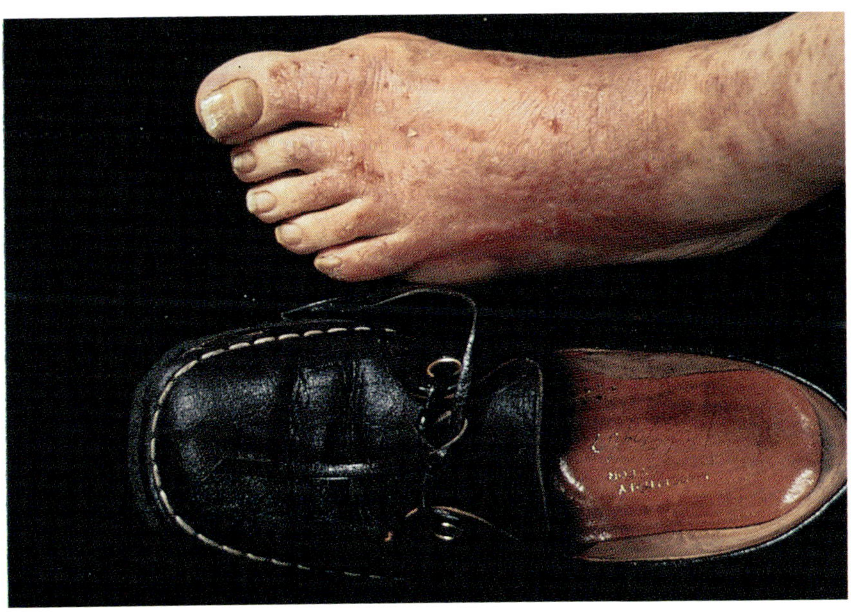

Courtesy of Donald V. Belsito, M.D.

SHOE TOP

SHOES *Continued*

Case IV

This patient had a chronic foot dermatosis variously diagnosed as psoriasis, tinea, and eczema (*D*). Patch tests to the shoe sole lining and to rubber chemicals were positive.

Case V

This patient had acute, severe dermatitis of the soles of his feet (*E*). After symptomatic therapy and treatment with prednisone, the lesions resolved. The patient was patch tested and found positive to the lining of the shoe and to ethyl thiourea, present in one brand of running shoe.

RESOLUTION

All patients discovered that their lesions cleared after the diagnosis of shoe dermatitis was made and the offending materials were avoided. For several patients, however, it took weeks to months for clearing because of the chronic dermatitis. Shoe dermatitis often is a self-perpetuating eczema—status eczematicus. For this reason, it is sometimes necessary to prescribe extra supportive care such as prednisone and to have them wear hypoallergenic sandals for weeks to months.

CLINICAL COMMENTS

Shoe dermatitis was far more common in the past than it is at present. It is uncertain why its frequency appears to be decreasing; perhaps the shoe industry is more aware of the possible allergens in their products.

Rubber allergens are the most common allergens. Chromium in tanning solutions and chromium dyes occasionally are responsible, as are plastics rarely.

It is important to patch test these patients with the routine patch test series. If the patient tests negative to the rubber chemicals and other shoe allergens described above, one should then test with small pieces of the shoe taken from the part of the shoe that is in contact with the dermatitis. This can be done by cutting up the shoe or obtaining the material using a sharp, heavy curette. It is important that the test material is thin, since a pressure reaction could result if a thick piece of material is used.

The physician should always offer the patient allergen alternatives, as described by Fisher.

Reference

Fisher AA: Contact Dermatitis, 3rd ed. Philadelphia, Lea & Febiger, 1986, pp 283–337.

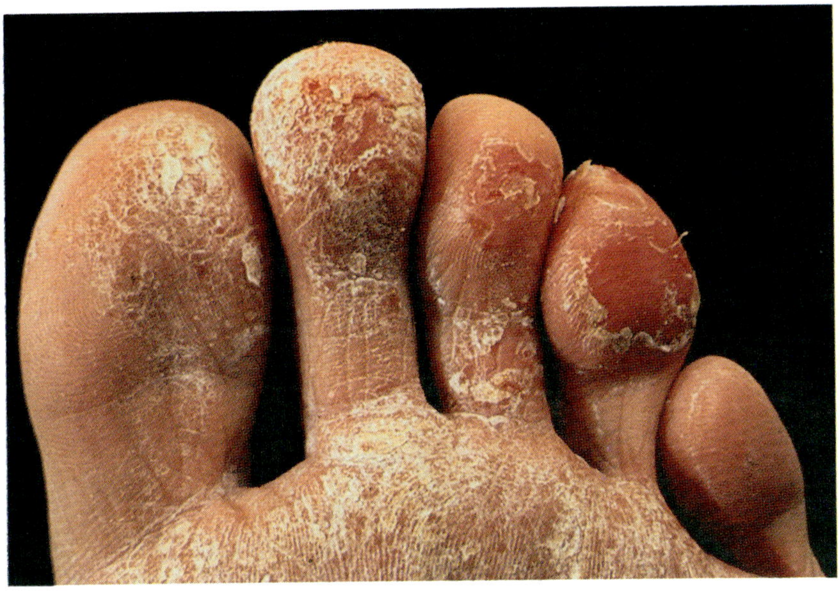

Courtesy of Donald V. Belsito, M.D.

SHOE LINING

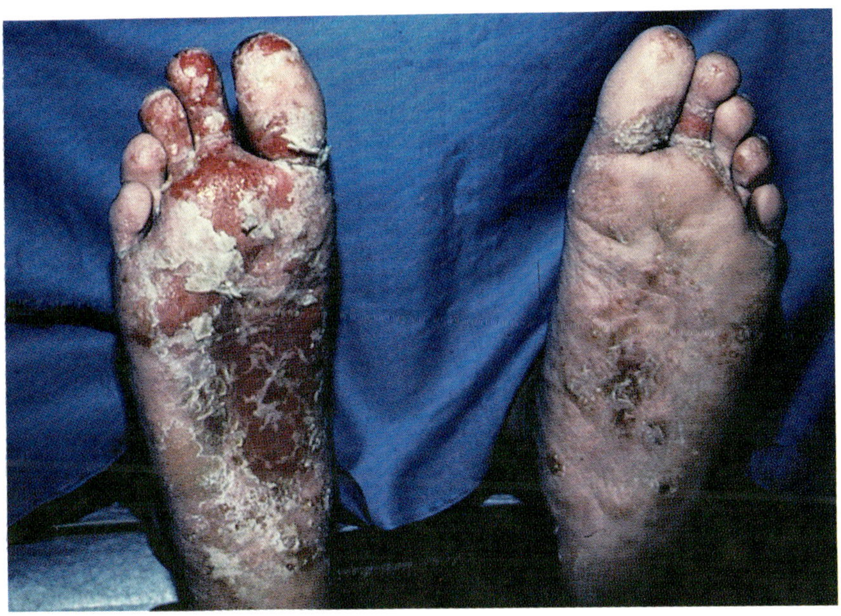

Courtesy of Donald V. Belsito, M.D.

RUNNING SHOES

MILKING MACHINE APPLIANCE

HISTORY

This farmer developed dermatitis that was insidious in onset and chronic in nature. Patch testing to the routine test series revealed a positive reaction to black rubber mix.

RESOLUTION

Subsequently, the farmer identified a rubber-containing milking machine appliance with which he had frequent contact. The chronic dermatitis resolved on discontinuing use of this instrument.

RUBBER GLOVES

HISTORY

A patient had chronic hand eczema. A recent exacerbation led to patch testing. The routine test series demonstrated a positive reaction to thiuram. Patch testing to the patient's rubber gloves was positive.

RESOLUTION

The dermatitis rapidly improved when the rubber gloves that the patient was using were replaced by heavy duty vinyl gloves. Thiuram-free rubber gloves are also available.

CLINICAL COMMENTS

Health care workers are using gloves with increasing frequency due to the AIDS epidemic. This has resulted in a resurgence of rubber glove reactions. Rich and co-workers list gloves that rubber-sensitive people can wear.

Reference

Rich P, Belozer ML, Norris P, Storrs FJ: Allergic contact dermatitis to two antioxidants in latex gloves: 4,4′-thiobis(6-tert-butyl-meta-cresol) (Lowinox 44S36) and butylhydroxyanisole. Allergen alternatives for glove-allergic patients. J Am Acad Dermatol 24(1):37–43, 1991.

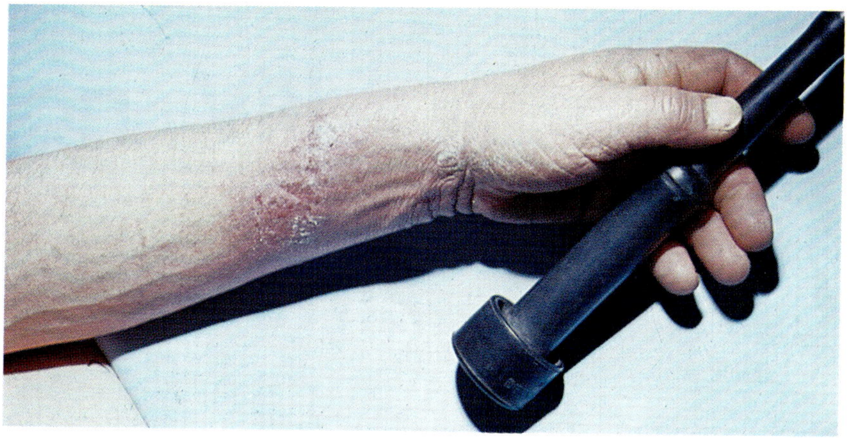

Courtesy of Frances J. Storrs, M.D.

MILKING MACHINE APPLIANCE

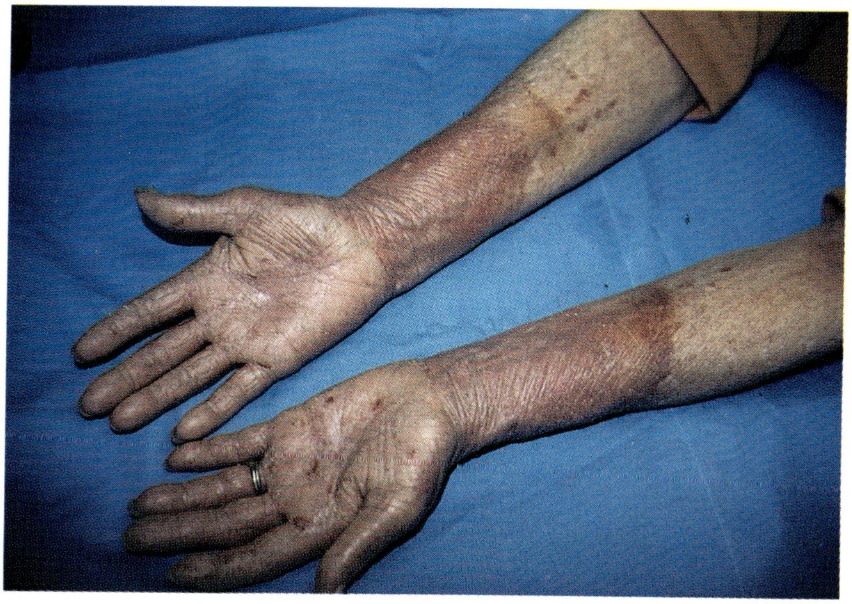

RUBBER GLOVES

BAG BALM

HISTORY

This patient had chronic hand eczema. The patch test noted here revealed a strong positive reaction to oxyquinolone. The dermatologist then reviewed the materials used by the patient, observing that in this case the product (Bag Balm) contained oxyquinolone. The routine test series produced a weak positive reaction to iodochlorhydroxyquin (Vioform).

RESOLUTION

The patient's hand eczema greatly improved but did not completely clear on removing the oxyquinolone exposure (Bag Balm).

CLINICAL COMMENTS

Medicament dermatitis is not always discovered using the routine test series. Vigilance is necessary in identifying the medicaments used by each patient.

Fortunately, most but not all, medicaments can be tested "as is" (undiluted) from the container, because most are formulated with low irritancy potential.

Reference

Breit R, Bandmann J-J: Contact dermatitis XXIV. The wide world of antimycotics. Br J Dermatol 89:657, 1973.

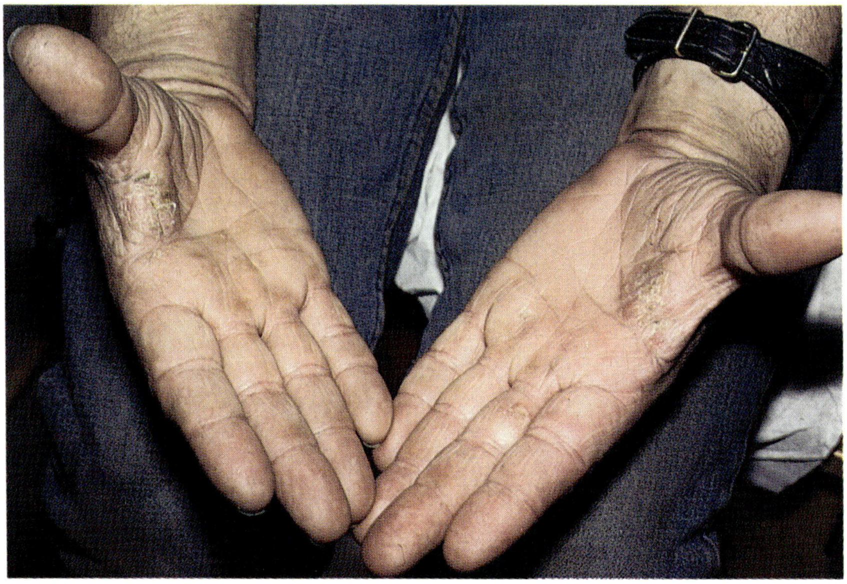

Courtesy of Frances J. Storrs, M.D.

BAG BALM DERMATITIS

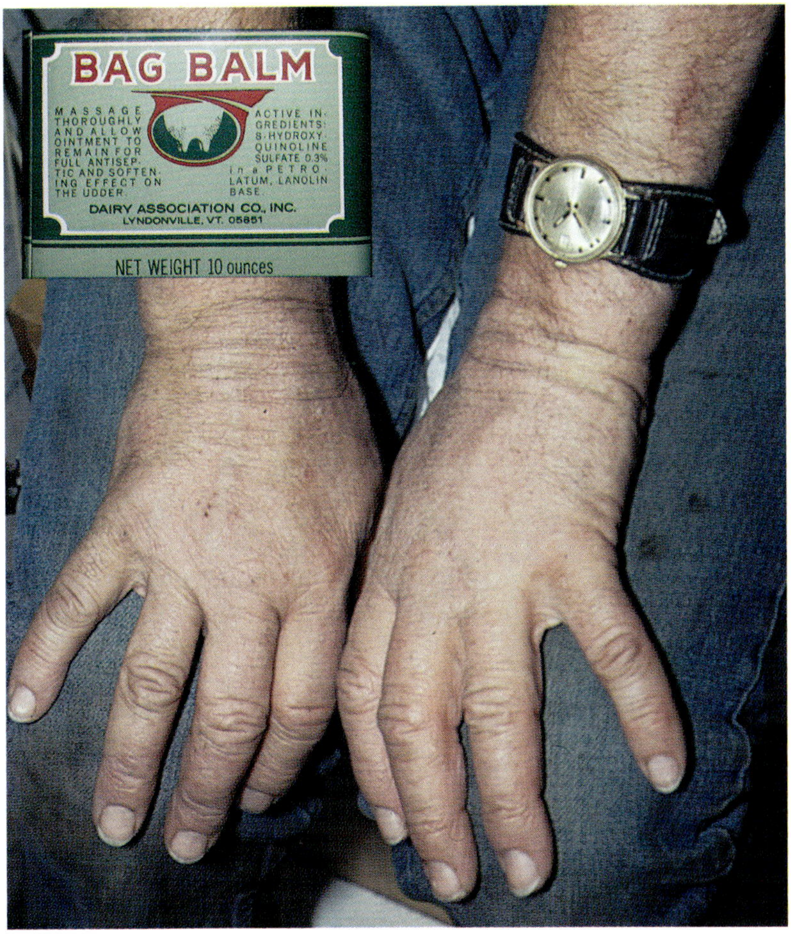

Courtesy of Frances J. Storrs, M.D.

BAG BALM DERMATITIS AND CONTAINER

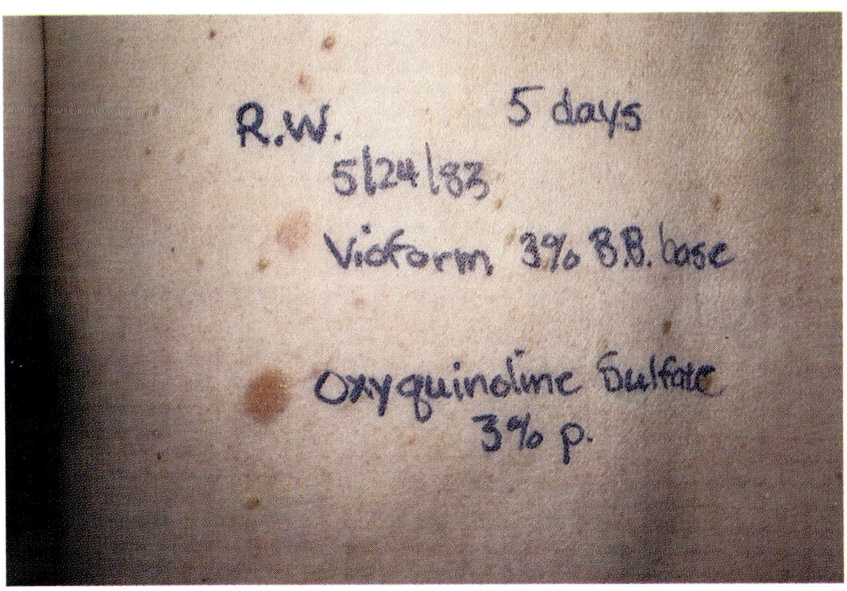

Courtesy of Frances J. Storrs, M.D.

BAG BALM PATCH TEST REACTIONS

TOPICAL CORTICOSTEROIDS

HISTORY

A patient had chronic eyelid eczema for which topical corticosteroids were prescribed. Because of chronicity, the patient was patch tested. Testing to the routine test series was negative; a strong positive result was identified with fluocinonide.

RESOLUTION

When the patient discontinued the use of this topical corticosteroid, the eczema rapidly and almost completely improved.

CLINICAL COMMENTS

Corticosteroid allergy is probably far more frequent than is generally appreciated. Recent large studies from Europe have revealed many individual allergens in corticosteroids. At the moment it is uncertain how to screen for topical steroid allergy. Certain marker substances such as hydrocortisone butyrate and tixocortol pivolate have been recommended. These are not commercially available patch test allergens. Furthermore, individual corticosteroid allergy may involve both the corticosteroid and some component in the vehicle.

The corticosteroids do not all cross react. For this reason, we test each patient with the corticosteroids they use. Unfortunately, there are often false negative test results with certain corticosteroids such as hydrocortisone; these require a higher than usual concentration. This may be because an impurity may be involved. Only a high index of suspicion will help identify such patients.

References

Dooms Gossens A: Allergic contact dermatitis to topical corticoids. Contact Dermatitis, *in press*.
Sasaki E: Corticosteroid sensitivity and cross-sensitivity. Contact Dermatitis 23:306–315, 1990.

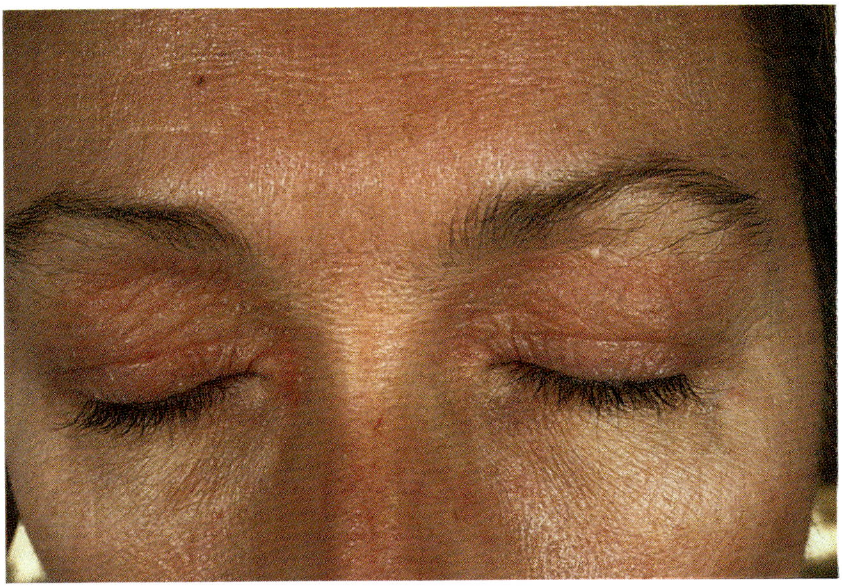

Courtesy of Donald V. Belsito, M.D.

CORTICOSTEROID CREAM DERMATITIS

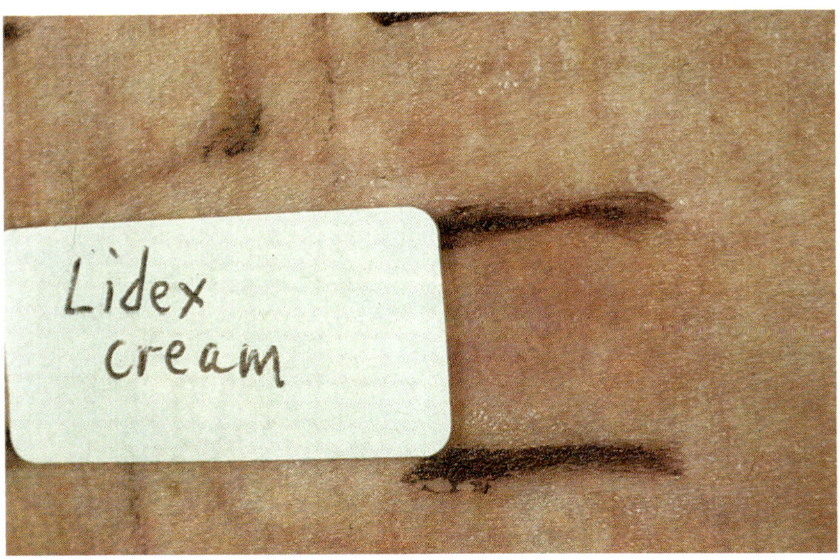

Courtesy of Donald V. Belsito, M.D.

FLUOCINONIDE PATCH TEST REACTION

FLUOCINONIDE

HISTORY

A 21-year-old university student with chronic hand eczema used a potent topical corticosteroid under plastic glove occlusion nightly, and often during the day, for 8 months. Gradually pigment was lost in selected areas. Following treatment cessation, her pigmentation gradually returned.

RESOLUTION

Repigmentation was slow and caused the patient considerable frustration and embarrassment, but with encouragement by her physician, she applied only bland hand creams to her hands and also avoided excessive sunlight during the repigmentation course. After about 8 months, pigmentation had returned to normal.

CLINICAL COMMENTS

Atrophy following excessive and prolonged use of topical corticosteroids is well known. Loss of pigment is also a complication of use of these potent medications, and of course it is more noticeable in patients with a greater degree of pigmentation.

References

Fisher AA: Contact Dermatitis, 3rd ed. Philadelphia, Lea & Febiger, 1986, p 679.
Suber C, Maibach H: Topical Corticosteroids. New York, Thomas Karger, 1991.

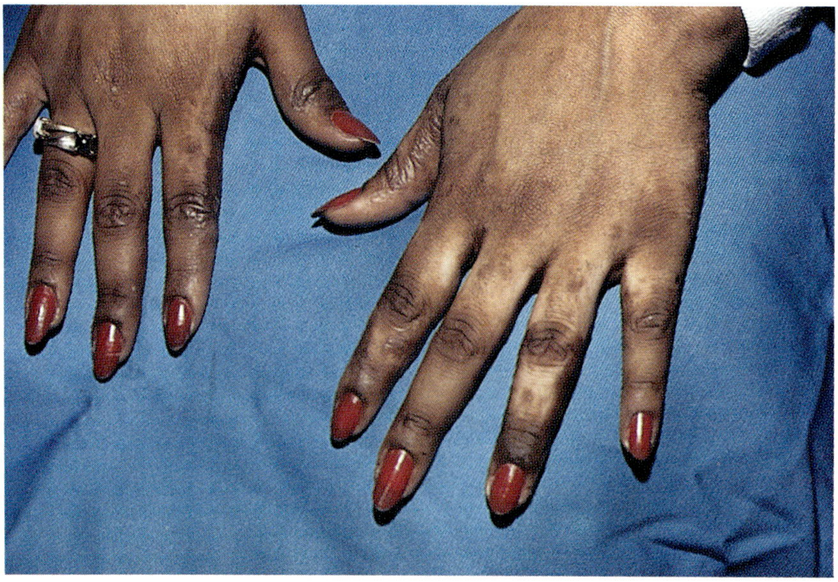

FLUOCINONIDE HYPOPIGMENTATION

Section IX

Dental Materials

SCOPOLAMINE

HISTORY

For over 4 years, this patient intermittently had used transdermal scopolamine for amelioration of motion sickness. Subsequently, each use produced a pruritic dermatitis consisting of erythema and induration.

RESOLUTION

Patch testing showed a positive reaction to scopolamine 1% in petrolatum. The patient was advised to discontinue use of scopolamine in transdermal form.

CLINICAL COMMENTS

Allergen alternative consists in the use of oral scopolamine.

Reference

Hogan D, Maibach H: Adverse dermatologic reactions to transdermal drug delivery systems. J Am Acad Dermatol 22:811–814, 1990.

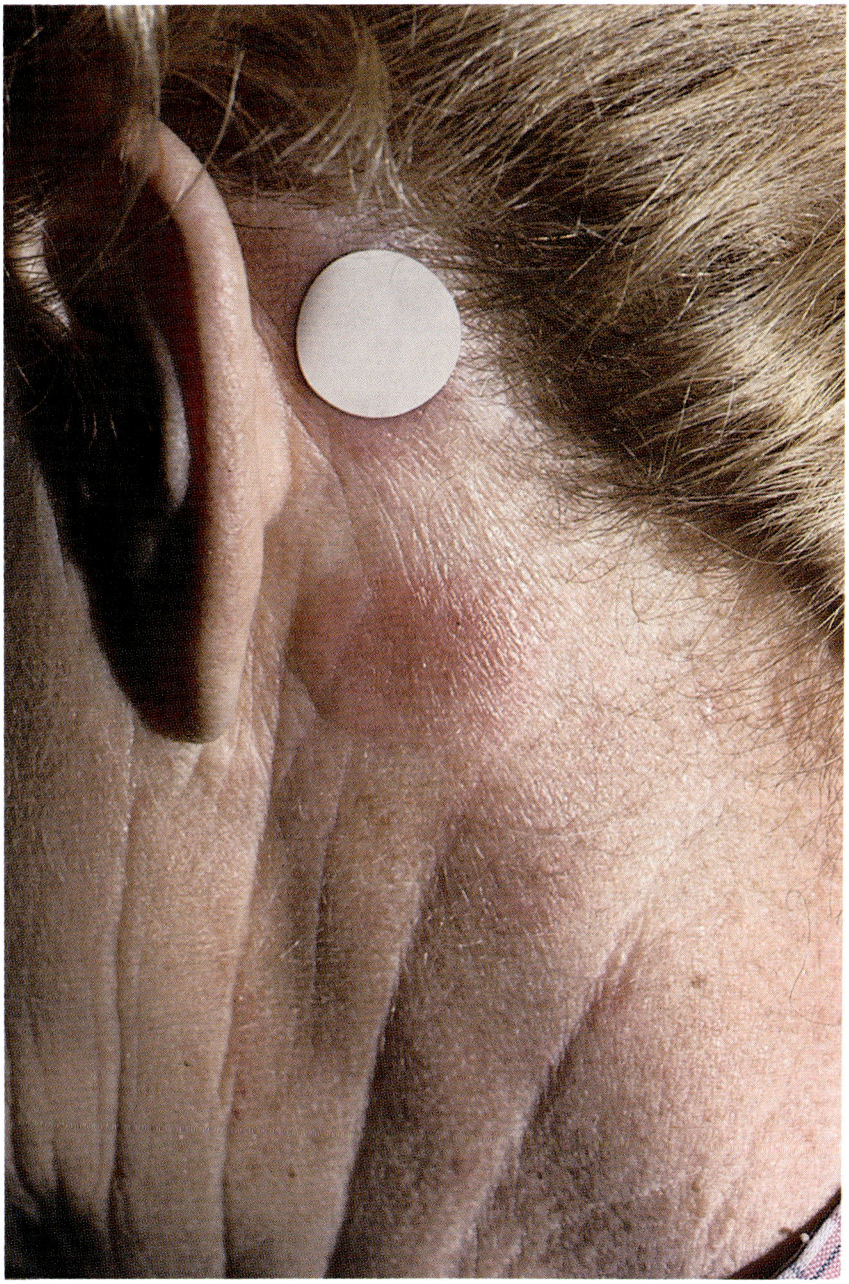

SCOPOLAMINE

Section XII

Miscellaneous

GARLIC

HISTORY

A 33-year-old man whose hobby was cooking developed a persistent, pruritic, scaling dermatitis on the volar aspect of the left distal thumb and the index and third fingers. Painful fissures developed intermittently. The history revealed he was right handed and held pieces of garlic in his left hand between the tips of these fingers while slicing. Patch testing to the juice of the garlic, 5% in petrolatum, revealed a strong positive reaction.

RESOLUTION

Using a garlic press, or employing only powdered garlic while cooking, resulted in disappearance of the dermatitis.

CLINICAL COMMENT

The allergen in garlic is thought to be diallyl disulfide, but it is not yet commercially available for patch testing. This substance is irritating and should be tested at 5% in petrolatum. Avoid testing with undiluted pieces of garlic, because the spice is highly irritating.

References

Adams RM: Food preparation workers. In Adams RM (ed): Occupational Skin Disease, 2nd ed. Philadelphia, WB Saunders, 1990, pp 623–625.
Hausen BM, Hjorth N: Skin reactions to topical food exposures. Dermatol Clin North Am 2:571, 1984.

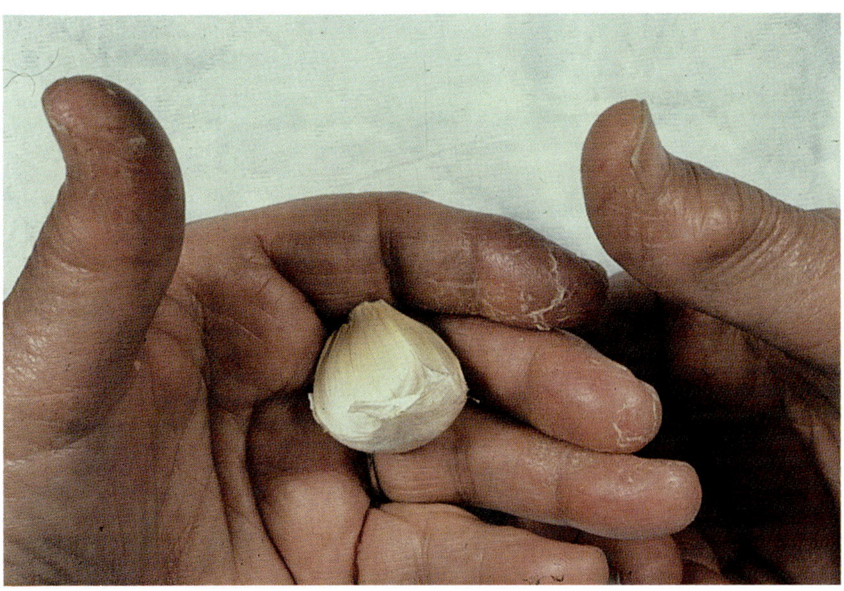

Courtesy of Donald V. Belsito, M.D.

GARLIC

JEANS BUTTON

HISTORY

This woman developed an eruption around her umbilicus that was initially diagnosed as a fungus infection. Later the eruption was found to be due to allergic sensitivity to nickel in the button of her blue jeans.

RESOLUTION

By eliminating contact between the button and the skin, the eruption disappeared. Application of clear nail polish or Varathane to the button may be used to coat the offending metal and will sometimes prevent recurrence.

CLINICAL COMMENTS

Nickel is a very common contact allergen, chiefly in women. Some are so exquisitely sensitive that even the small amount of nickel in coins will induce an eruption.

The use of the dimethylglyoximine test for determining the presence of nickel is indispensable in management of nickel dermatitis. Nickel-sensitive patients can be instructed in use of this test and avoid further dermatitis.

Some patients with blue jeans button dermatitis are primarily sensitized with the nickel in the button and not from previous jewelry nickel.

Brandrup and Larsen examined 79 nickel-sensitive patients and found that about 65% of them had had eczema due to metallic buttons.

Some nickel-sensitive patients react to 0.5 ppm nickel sulfate on slightly dermatitic skin. This new information will greatly alter our management of nickel allergic contact dermatitis patients.

Reference

Brandrup F, Larsen FS: Nickel dermatitis provoked by buttons in blue jeans. Contact Dermatitis 5:148, 1979.

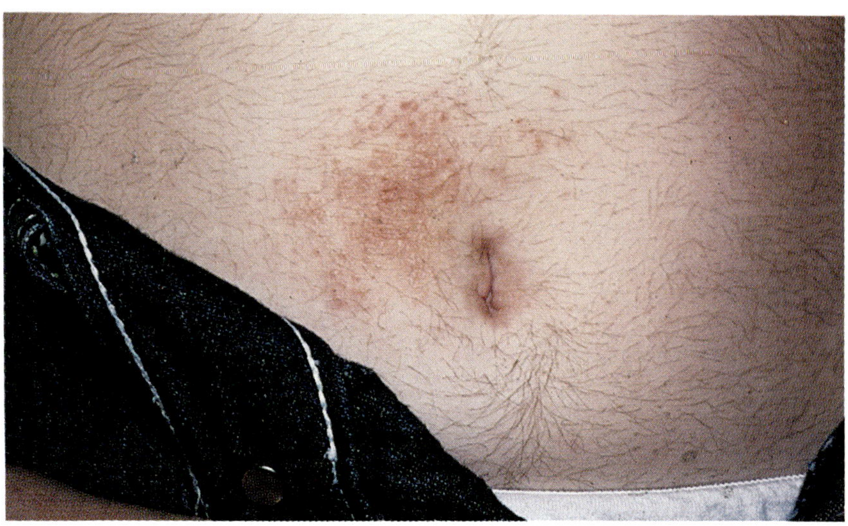

JEANS BUTTON

EYEGLASS FRAME

HISTORY

A 40-year-old airline pilot developed a persistent, pruritic dermatitis under the plastic of his glasses. The condition was especially annoying to him when on long-distance flights. It began shortly after purchasing a new pair of glasses with clear plastic frames. Patch testing to scrapings of the plastic frames and resorcinol monobenzoate 1% in petrolatum was positive at 72 and 96 hours.

RESOLUTION

Following purchase of a new pair of glasses with clear plastic frames manufactured by a different company, the dermatitis subsided.

CLINICAL COMMENT

Resorcinol monobenzoate is used as an ultraviolet inhibitor in clear plastics, especially cellulose esters, to prevent yellowish discoloration. Not all clear plastics used in manufacture of eyeglass frames contain this substance, however, and it is rarely if ever used in those manufactured in the United States. Because the chemical is an ingredient of balsam of Peru, patch test reactions to this allergen are frequently found. Resorcinol monobenzoate is now available commercially for patch testing.

References

Jordan WP Jr: Resorcinol monobenzoate, steering wheels, Peruvian balsam. Arch Dermatol 108:278, 1973.

Jordan WP, Dahl MV: Contact dermatitis from cellulose ester plastics. Arch Dermatol 105:880, 1972.

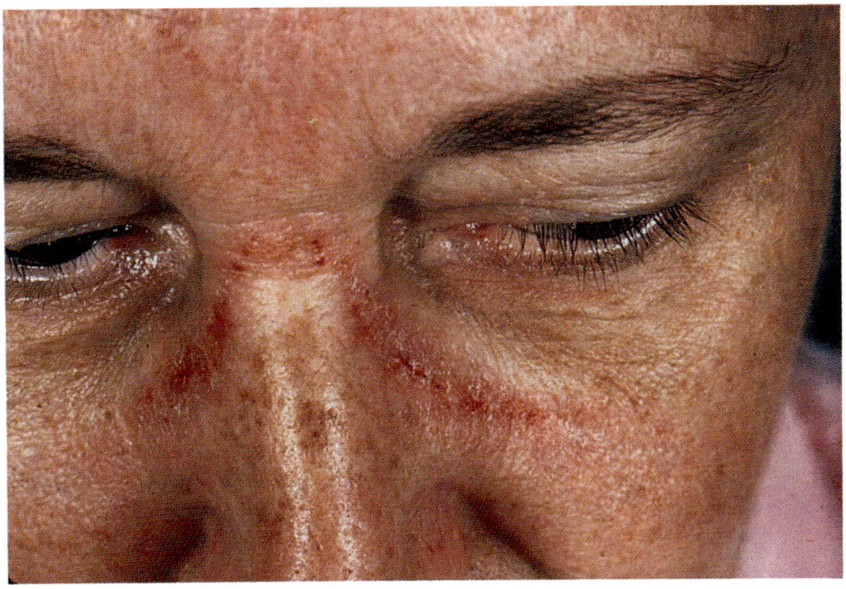

Courtesy of Donald V. Belsito, M.D.

EYEGLASS FRAME

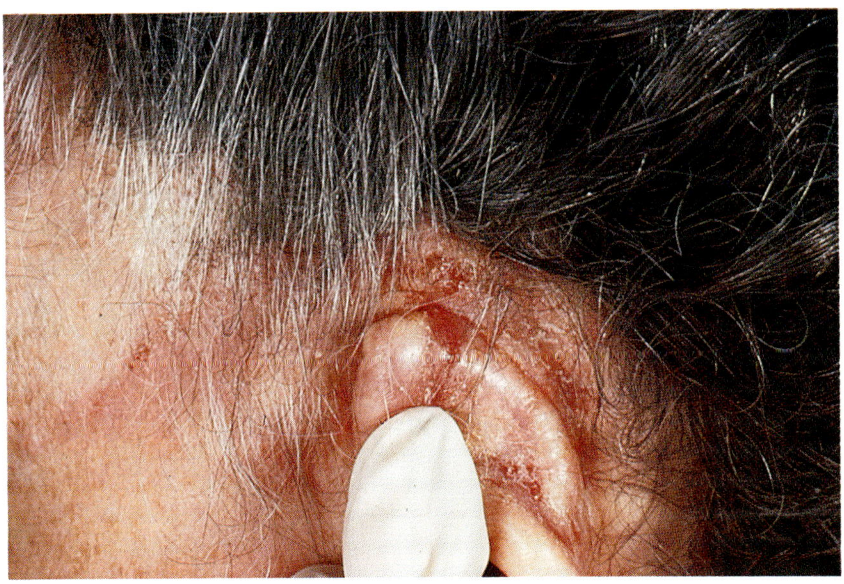

Courtesy of Donald V. Belsito, M.D.

EYEGLASS FRAME

COLOR FILM DEVELOPER

HISTORY

A photographic worker developed an eruption on the hands and arms after working with color film developers CD3 and CD4. Biopsy showed spongiosus and a lichenoid infiltrate.

RESOLUTION

The eruption cleared promptly following automation of the photographic process, but recurrences may develop when the patient is cleaning and repairing the developer.

CLINICAL COMMENTS

Photographic workers develop this peculiar lichen planus-like eruption from CD3 and CD4, chemicals that are derivatives of p-phenylanadiamine and aniline. This reaction may also occur in amateur photographers.

Reference

Knudsen E: Lichen planus-like eruption caused by color developer. Arch Dermatol 89:357, 1964.

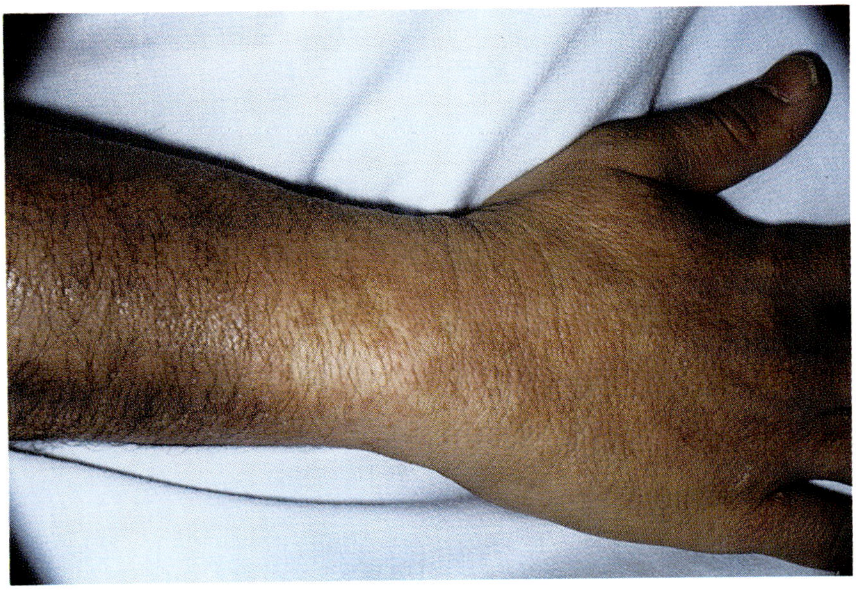

Courtesy of Ronald R. Brancaccio, M.D.

COLOR FILM DEVELOPER DERMATITIS

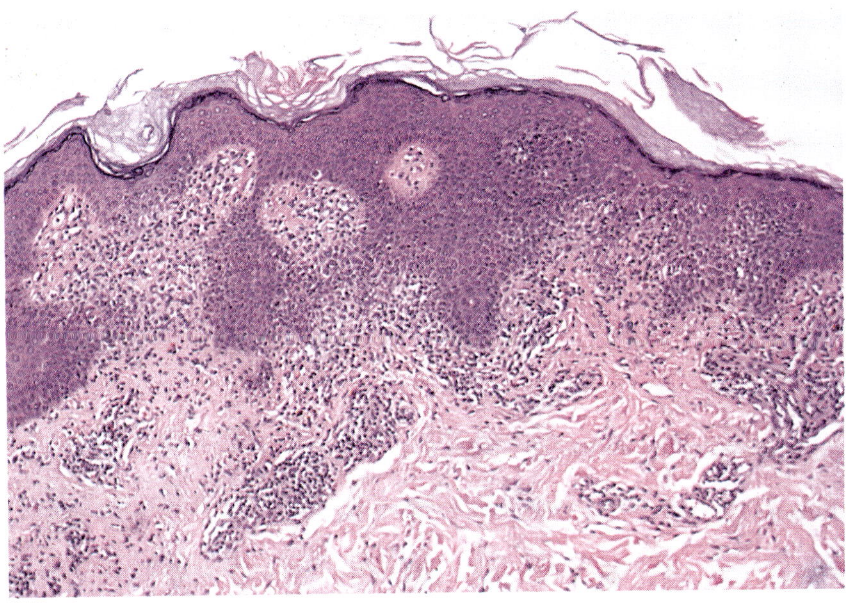

Courtesy of Ronald R. Brancaccio, M.D.

COLOR FILM DEVELOPER DERMATITIS BIOPSY

ACID PERMANENT WAVE

HISTORY

Every 3 months this 29-year-old woman has a permanent wave in a beauty salon. A highly pruritic rash developed 24 hours after the latest permanent, which was heat-cured. Patch testing to glyceryl monothioglycolate 1% in petrolatum was strongly positive.

RESOLUTION

By requesting that the beauty salon operator use only the older ammonium thioglycolate for permanents, this woman was able to avoid recurrence. The dermatitis persisted for several weeks, however.

CLINICAL COMMENTS

The so-called "acid perms" containing glyceryl monothioglycolate today account for more than 50% of permanents used in beauty salons. They are considered more effective than the old alkaline permanents based on ammonium thioglycolate. The operator is usually the person sensitized, but clients also are at risk. The allergen remains on the hair for up to 3 months, and thus sensitized individuals may experience recurring dermatitis for long periods. Because the allergen readily passes through latex gloves, sensitized operators may be forced to change occupations. 4H gloves are protective (Accaderm Co., Menlo Park, CA). The allergen in petrolatum is unstable and should be renewed approximately every 6 months.

References

Morrison LH, Storrs FJ: Persistence of an allergen in hair after glyceryl monothioglycolate-containing permanent wave solutions. J Am Acad Dermatol 19:52–59, 1988.

Storrs FJ: Permanent wave contact dermatitis: Contact allergy to glyceryl monothioglycolate. J Am Acad Dermatol 11:74–85, 1984.

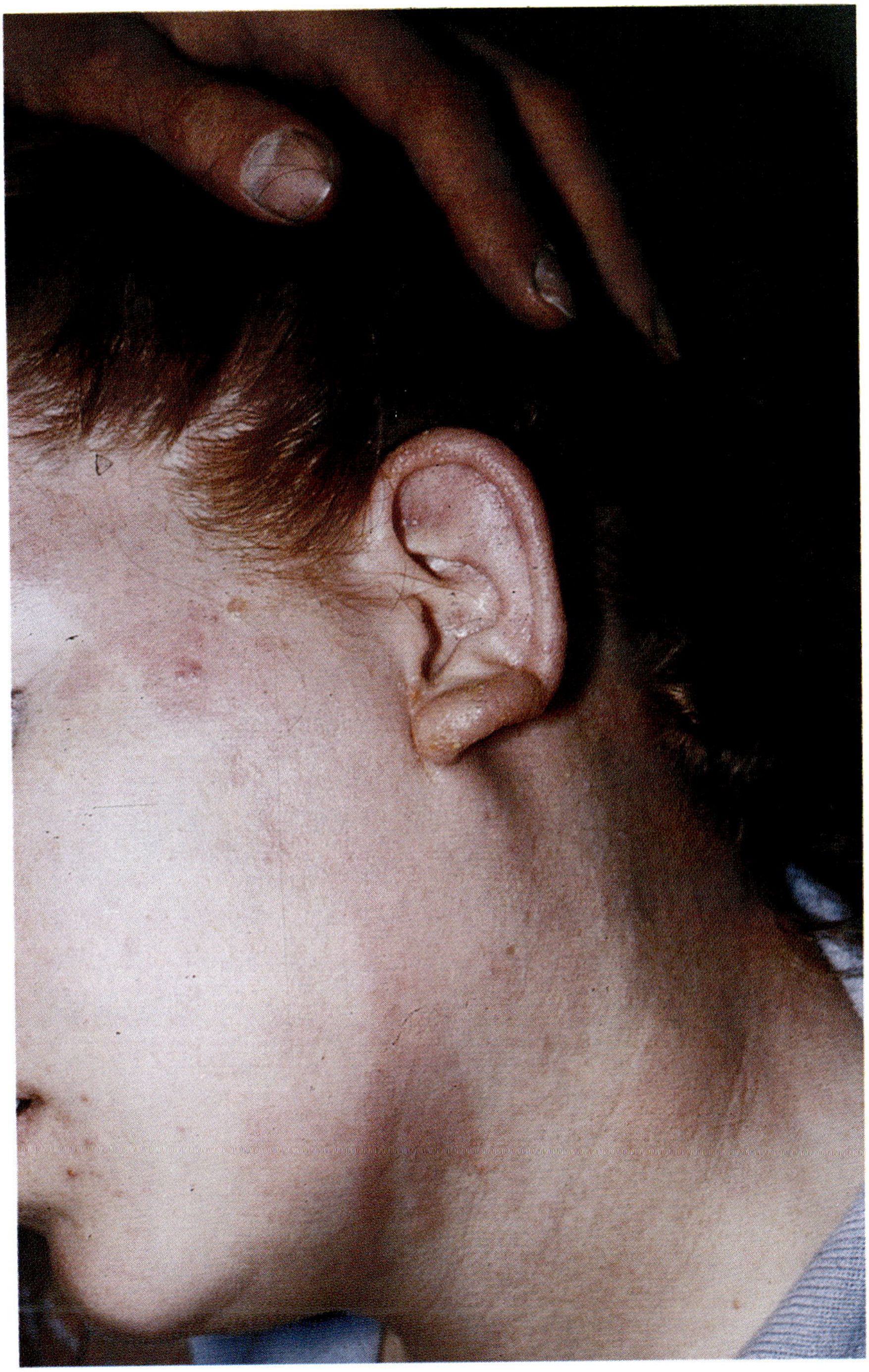

Courtesy of Frances J. Storrs, M.D.

PERMANENT WAVE

COPY PAPER

HISTORY

A 52-year-old draftsman developed pruritic dermatitis and tiny blisters on his fingertips. The thumbs and first three fingers of both hands were most affected. Initially the dermatitis was thought to be constitutional, and a contact allergen at work was not suspected. Later, patch testing results were positive to unexposed blueprint paper as well as to the diazonium dyes p-aminoazobenzene and p-diethylaminobenzene diazonium chloride, both 1% in petrolatum, which are related to the dyes used in the paper.

RESOLUTION

By wearing cloth gloves (as shown in the photograph), the draftsman was able to minimize recurrences. Because he was highly paid and had worked for his company for more than 20 years, he was reluctant to change occupations.

CLINICAL COMMENTS

Blueprint paper is sensitized with a diazonium salt and coupler, and an acid is present to prevent coupling before use. Exposure to ultraviolet light destroys the diazonium salt, and treatment with ammonia neutralizes the acid, causing the coupling reaction and the lines of the drawing to appear in blue against a white background. Most blueprint workers believe that ammonia is the cause of their dermatitis. Care must be taken to prevent exposing the paper to light prior to testing.

References

Conde Salazar L, Romero L, Guimaraens D: Allergic contact dermatitis from diazo paper. Contact Dermatitis 8:210–211, 1982.

Crijns MB, Boom BW, van der Schroeff JG: Allergic contact dermatitis to a diazonium compound in copy paper. Contact Dermatitis 16:112–113, 1987.

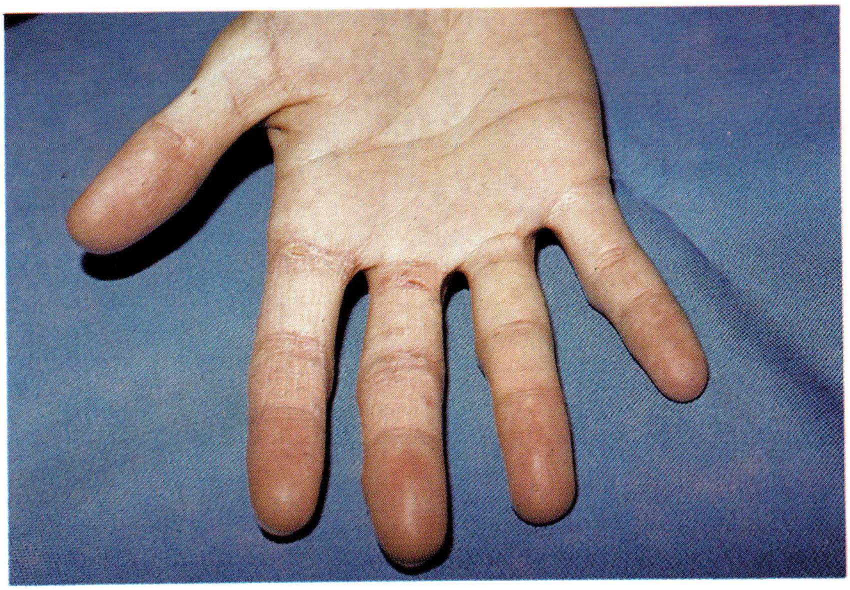

COPY PAPER DERMATITIS

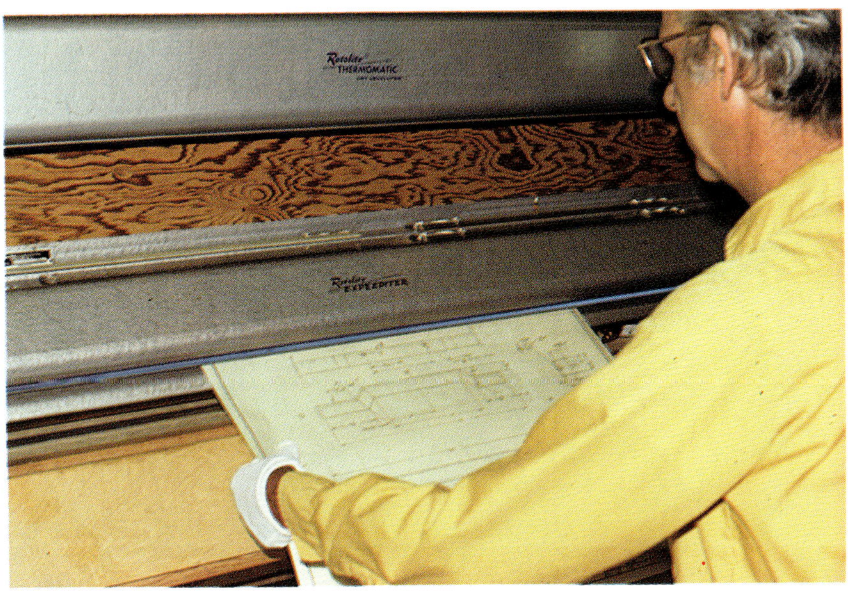

CLOTH GLOVES FOR COPY PAPER DERMATITIS

VITAMIN K

HISTORY

A nurse received an injection of vitamin K because of a spontaneous bleeding episode. Two weeks following the injection, dermatitis developed at the injection site. Patch testing to the product tested "as is" was positive at 48 hours.

RESOLUTION

Even with the use of topical corticosteroid creams, the reaction persisted for over 2 months.

CLINICAL COMMENTS

Vitamin K (Aquamephyton) is phytonadione. Delayed hypersensitivity to vitamin K is rare. Most vitamin K exposure occurs in workers manufacturing the substance.

Reference

Jirasek L: Hypersensitivity to vitamin K. Cesk Derm 40:17, 1965.

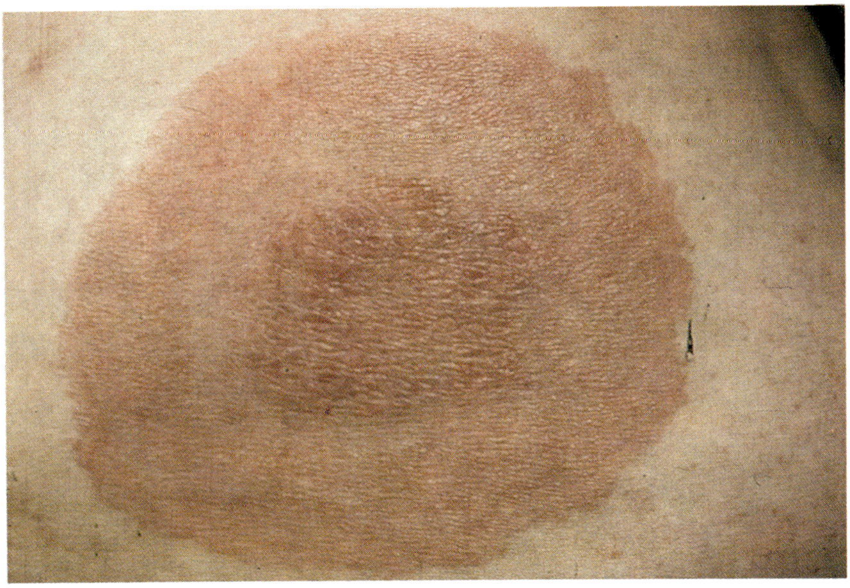

Courtesy of Ronald R. Brancaccio, M.D.

VITAMIN K DERMATITIS

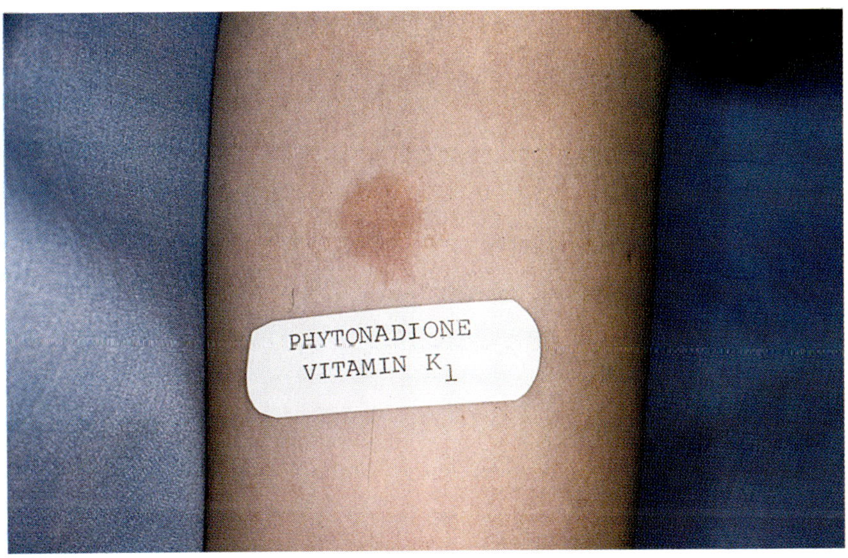

Courtesy of Ronald R. Brancaccio, M.D.

VITAMIN K PATCH TEST

COMPUTER MOUSE PAD

HISTORY

A computer operator developed an eruption on the thenar and hypothenar eminences of his right hand. History revealed that he used a computer with a "mouse" and a pad.

RESOLUTION

Substitution of a different brand of pad completely resolved the dermatitis.

CLINICAL COMMENTS

This case emphasizes the importance of morphology and a thorough history. With the widespread use of computers with "mouse" pads, this type of reaction may not be unusual.

Results of patch testing to the pad were negative, thus representing an irritant reaction.

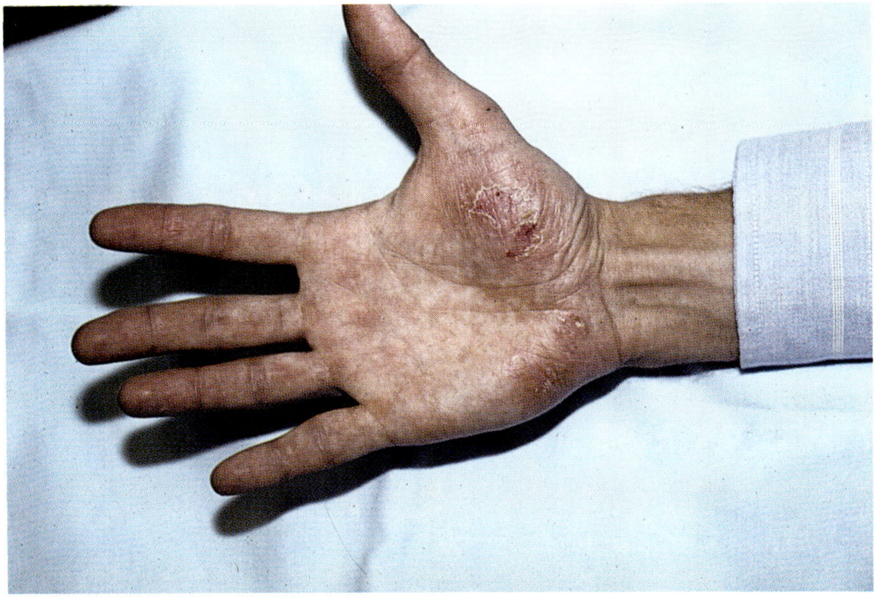

Courtesy of Robert Bell, M.D.

COMPUTER MOUSE PAD REACTION

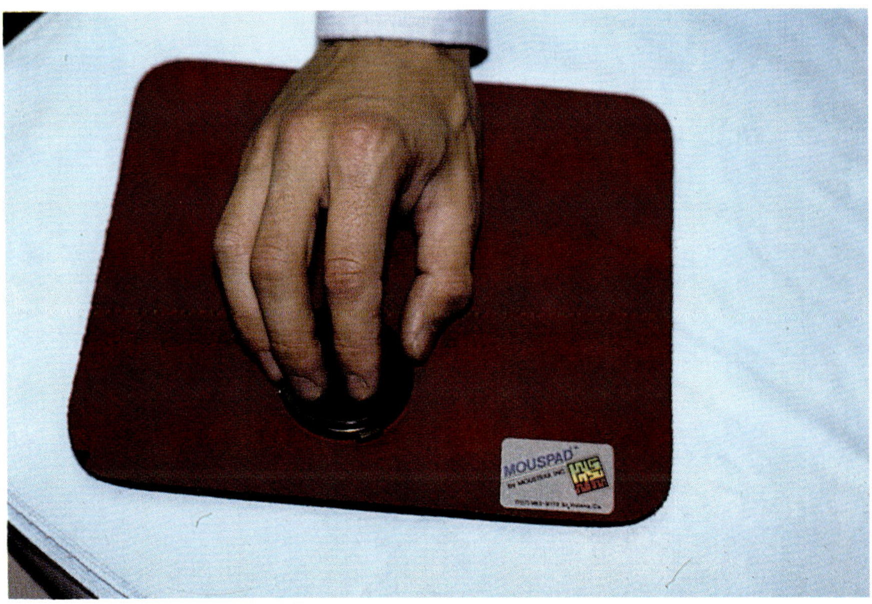

REPLACEMENT PAD

FIRE CORAL

HISTORY

This man developed an unusual eruption on the left side of his chest after snorkeling in the Bahamas, where he inadvertently brushed against fire coral.

RESOLUTION

The eruption cleared promptly with the use of a potent topical corticosteroid cream.

CLINICAL COMMENTS

Tropical fire coral is a stinging coral that produces an erythematous, burning lesion due to a high concentration of formic acid. Fire coral is yellowish-brown in color and located on most tropical reefs.

Stinging or fire coral dermatitis is not caused by a coral but by a nematocyst living on the wet mucus of the organism *Millepora alcincornis*. Fire coral lives among true coral throughout tropical oceans, such as the Caribbean Sea. The eruption, thought to be caused by a high concentration of formic acid, usually subsides in 2 or 3 days.

References

Fisher AA: Atlas of Aquatic Dermatology. New York, Grune & Stratton, 1978, pp 20–21.
Fisher AA: Contact Dermatitis, 3rd ed. Philadelphia, Lea & Febiger, 1986, pp 808–810.

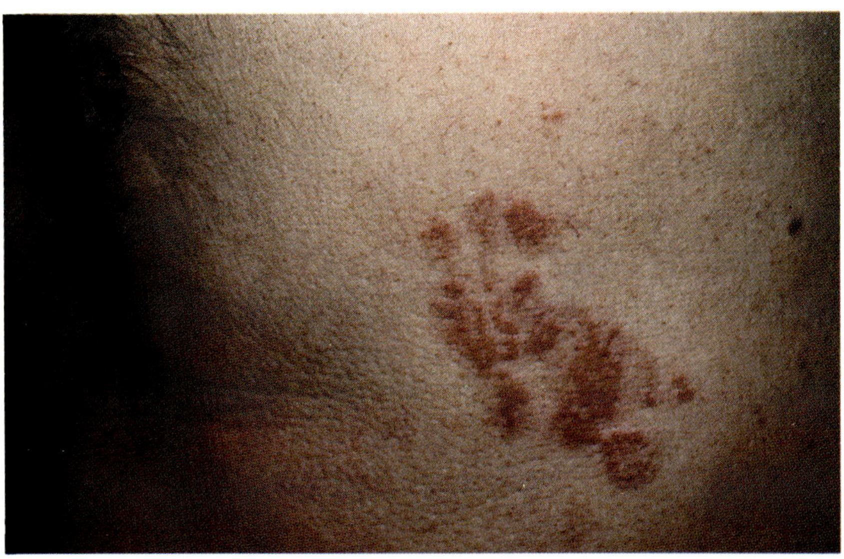

FIRE CORAL

Section XIII

Mimics of Contact Dermatitis

TINEA AS A "POSITIVE PATCH TEST"

HISTORY

This woman presented with what was thought to be contact dermatitis of the feet due to shoes (*A*). Patch testing on the arm from two parts of the shoe resulted in positive reactions (*B*). However, the reaction on the arm continued to expand and began to scale peripherally, and on scraping was found to be potassium hydroxide (KOH)-positive.

RESOLUTION

This patient did not have contact dermatitis but instead had tinea pedis. Patch testing to the shoe material provoked a false positive reaction, representing instead the transfer of fungi from shoe to arm. She responded rapidly to antifungal therapy.

CLINICAL COMMENT

Contact dermatitis to footwear and tinea infection of the feet can sometimes be difficult to differentiate. This case demonstrates the value of a KOH examination of the feet and a culture for fungal elements.

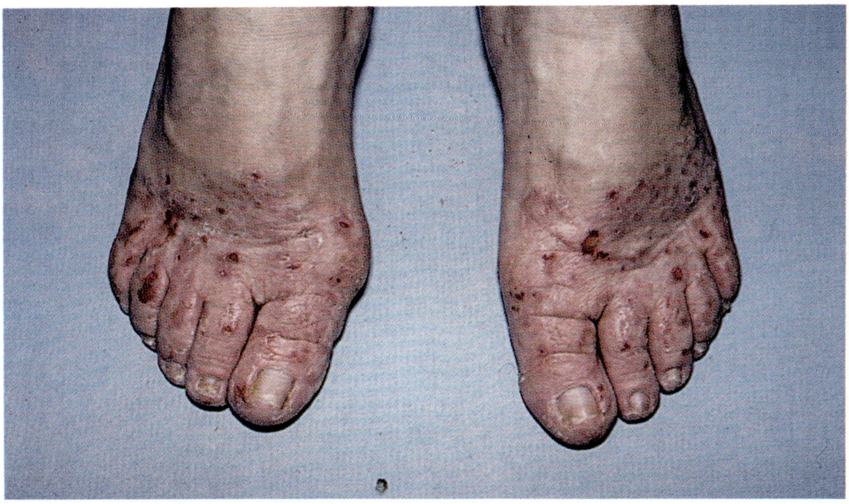

Courtesy of William P. Jordan, M.D.

TINEA PEDIS

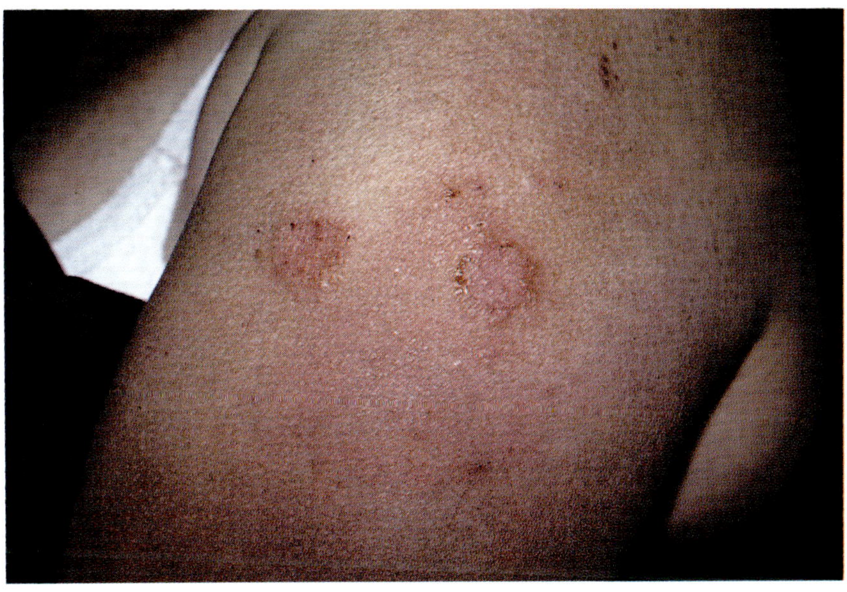

Courtesy of William P. Jordan, M.D.

FALSE POSITIVE TINEA REACTION

CORTICOSTEROID DERMATITIS

HISTORY

For 6 months this 17-year-old girl applied a potent topical corticosteroid to her face for mild seborrhea. Gradually she noticed small "zits" accompanied by constant itching. The more "zits" she noticed, the more cream she applied. A disturbing decrease in pigment also was seen.

RESOLUTION

Discontinuance of the corticosteroid resulted in complete clearing of the acne-like condition in about 6 months; the pigment required several months longer to return.

CLINICAL COMMENTS

Corticosteroid acne and hypopigmentation are fairly common sequelae of long-term, intensive application of potent topical corticosteroids. Discontinuance results in return of previously normal skin but not until many months have elapsed.

Reference

Arnold HL, Odom RB, James WB: Andrews' Diseases of Skin, 8th ed. Philadelphia, WB Saunders, 1990, p 250.

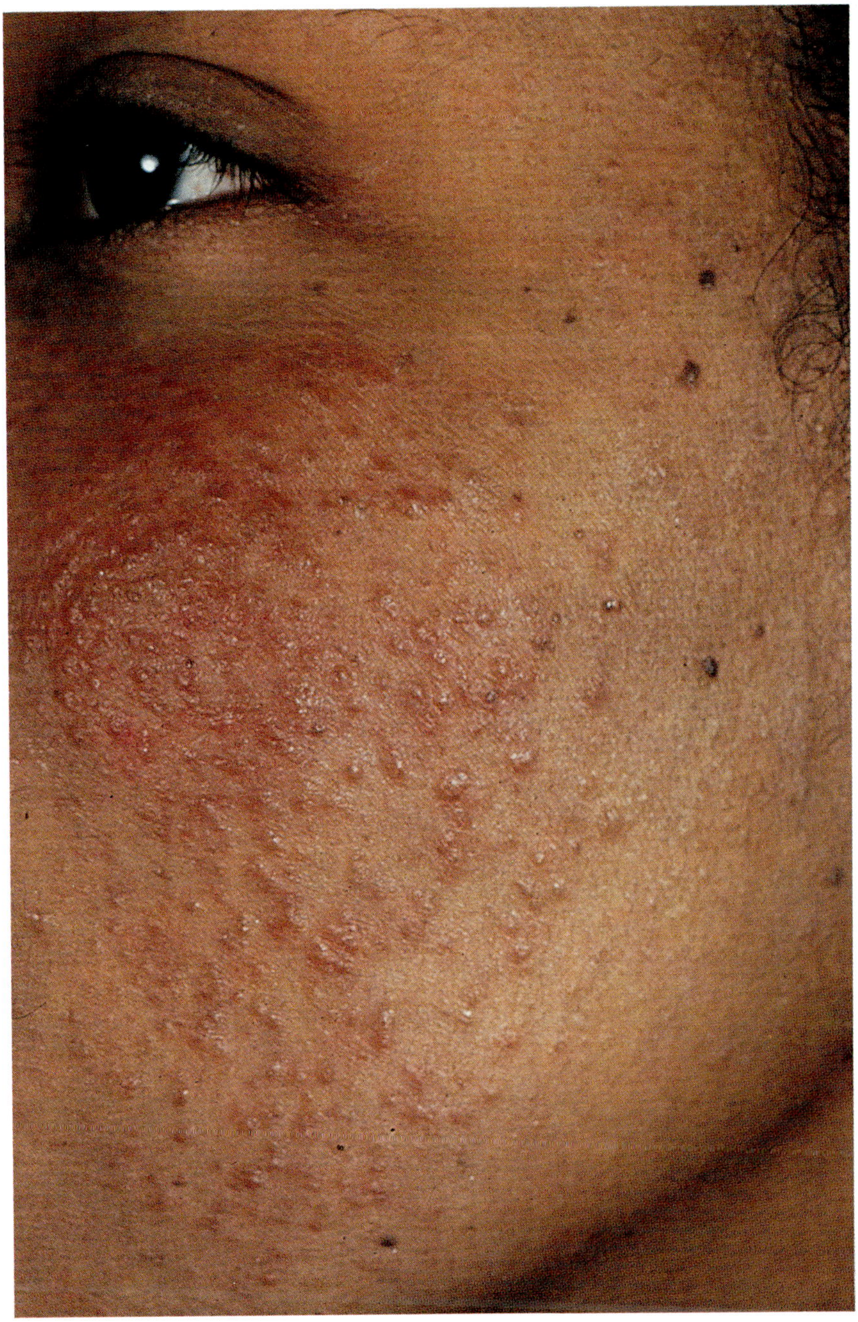

Courtesy of Donald V. Belsito, M.D.

STEROID CREAM

PSORIASIS

HISTORY

This condition developed rapidly on a 25-year-old mail carrier. Initially it was thought to be due to an allergic reaction to his shoes, but patch testing to standard patch test allergens, including small pieces of the inner sole of his shoes, revealed negative results. Biopsy supported a diagnosis of psoriasis.

Psoriasis on the palm is frequently mistaken for contact dermatitis.

RESOLUTION

The patient filed a worker compensation claim for psoriasis on his feet, which later appeared also on the hands and other areas. The claim was denied, although it appeared the work did indeed result in temporary aggravation of this presumably preexisting condition.

CLINICAL COMMENTS

In the usual case of psoriasis of the soles of the feet, there should be no difficulty in reaching a diagnosis of psoriasis. In patients in whom the appearance is atypical, however, the possibility of allergic contact dermatitis may be considered. Occasionally contact allergy and psoriasis are present jointly, in which case removal of the offending allergen can result in considerable improvement in the psoriasis.

Reference

Epstein E: Eczematous psoriasis. In Roenigk H, Maibach H (eds.): Psoriasis. New York, Marcel Dekker, 1991.

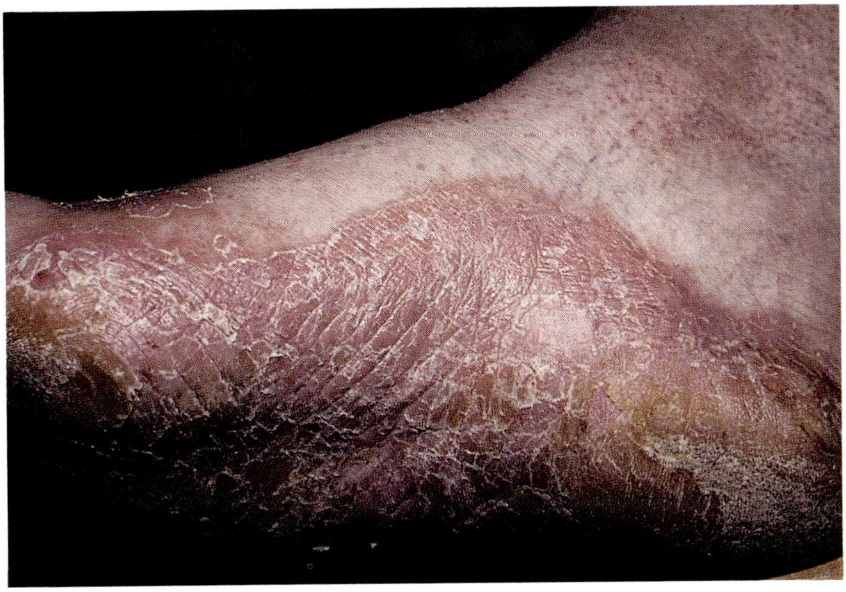

Courtesy of Frances J. Storrs, M.D.

PSORIASIS

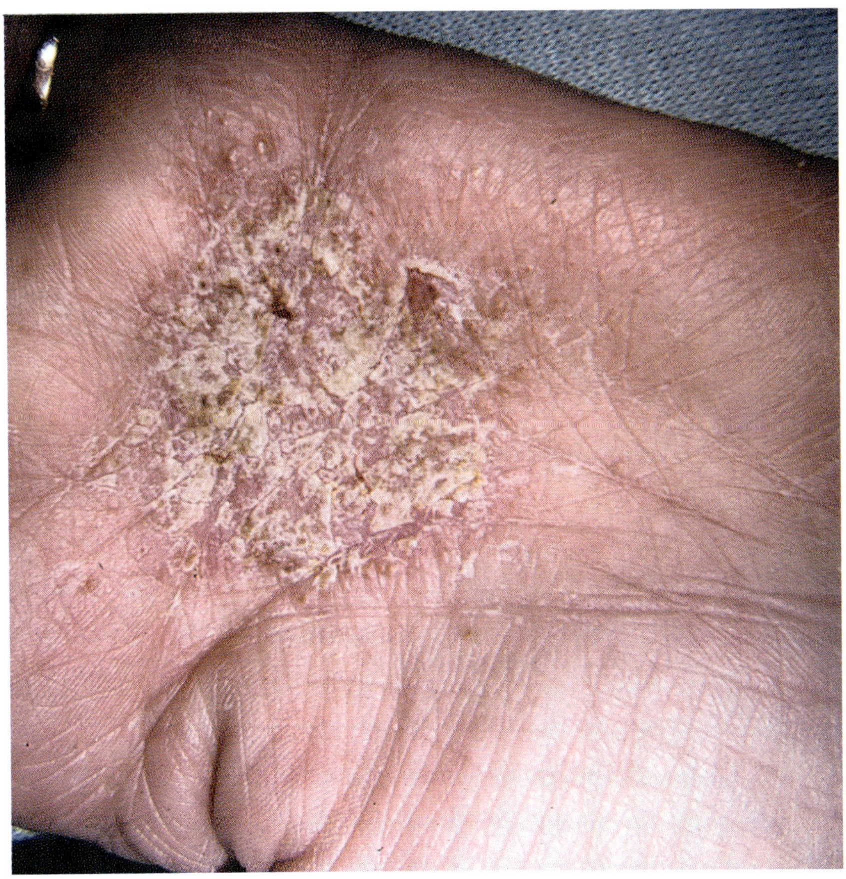

Courtesy of Alexander A. Fisher, M.D.

PSORIASIS

CHRONIC ECZEMA

HISTORY

Since age 17 this 52-year-old man has been employed as a stone mason. Approximately 2 years ago he noted the appearance of nonpruritic, hypertrophic scaling patches on his palms and fingers. Deep, painful fissures appear frequently on the volar tips of his fingers. At times the condition prevents his working.

RESOLUTION

Because pruritus was absent, patch testing was not considered. The appearance and patchy nature of the condition somewhat resemble that of contact dermatitis. Psoriasis also is important to consider in the differential diagnosis.

CLINICAL COMMENTS

This is a puzzling condition, often confused with psoriasis and allergic contact dermatitis. It can be extremely disabling and can cause severely affected workers to leave the workplace entirely. It improves somewhat when repeated friction ceases but recurs rapidly on return to work.

References

Adams RM: Occupational Skin Disease, 2nd ed. Philadelphia, WB Saunders, 1990, pp 203–214.
Epstein E: Eczematous psoriasis. In Roenigk H, Maibach H (eds): Psoriasis. New York, Marcel Dekker, 1991.

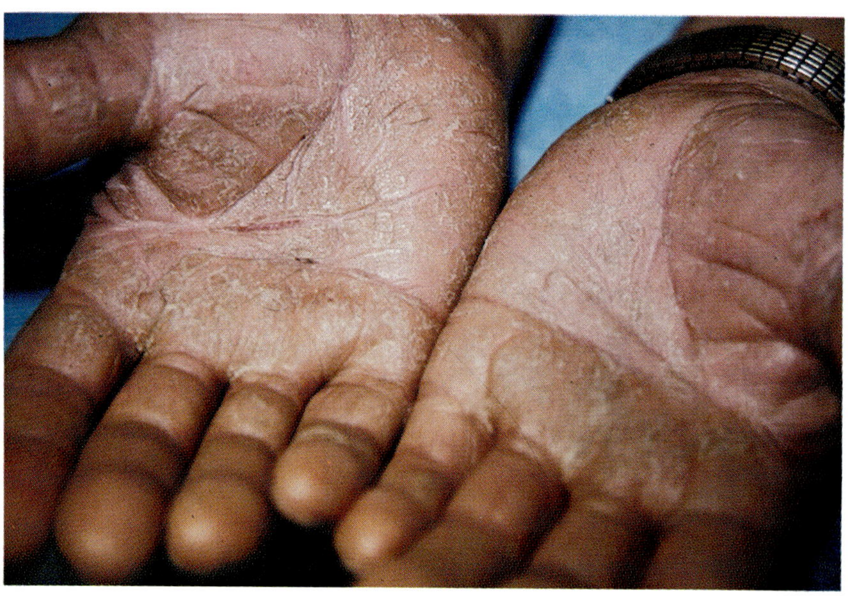

CHRONIC ECZEMA

SELF-INDUCED CONTACT DERMATITIS

HISTORY

Two and one-half months following a fractured wrist that occurred at work, a severely pruritic, eczematous dermatitis appeared on the dorsam of both hands but was more severe on the right. Biopsy showed acanthosis with areas of spongiosis, parakeratosis, and a mild mononuclear infiltrate in the dermis, findings consistent with contact dermatitis. Fungal smears and cultures were negative. Patch tests, including tests for medications, were negative. Treatment with various topical and systemic medications was of no avail, but application of an Unna dressing almost completely cleared the eruption on several occasions.

RESOLUTION

Treatment was of no benefit. The possibility of self-injury was suggested to the patient, which she vigorously denied. After this the patient was lost to followup.

CLINICAL COMMENT

Self-induced contact dermatitis is not common but is difficult to diagnose. One clue is the excessive nature of the reaction in relation to the possible causes. A thorough study is vital, leaving no possibility uncovered, however unlikely.

References

Fabisch W: Psychiatric aspects of dermatitis artefacta. Br J Dermatol 102:29, 1980.
Fisher BK, et al: Dermatitis artefacta. Cutis 19:665, 1977.
Koblenzer CS: Psychosomatic concepts in dermatology. Arch Dermatol 121:780, 1985.

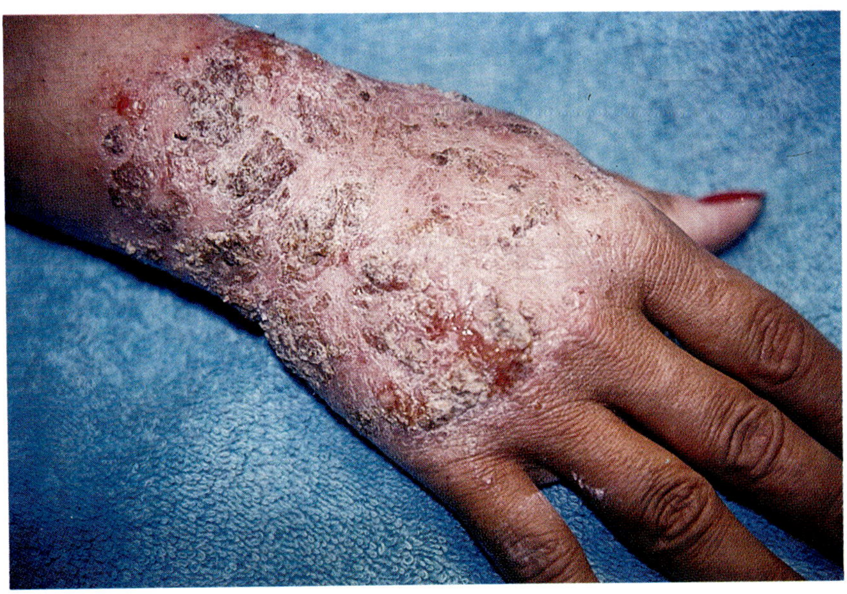

SELF-INDUCED CONTACT DERMATITIS

LICHEN SIMPLEX CHRONICUS

HISTORY

A 36-year-old Filipino farm worker presented for evaluation of the possible work relationship of a chronic, pruritic lesion of several years' duration on the lateral aspect of his right leg. No other skin areas were affected. The patient admitted to daily, prolonged rubbing of the area, often with a brush, usually with his knuckles. Patch testing requested by the insurance company was negative for standard and selected workplace allergens. Biopsy showed marked hyperkeratosis overlying an acanthotic epidermis with a mild lymphocytic infiltrate, indicating chronic dermatitis without clear evidence of psoriasis.

RESOLUTION

Treatment by the patient's local physician with topical corticoid ointments under occlusion resulted in clearing of the lesion. A new area of involvement appeared gradually on the right neck and at the nuchal area.

CLINICAL COMMENT

In most cases, lichen simplex chronicus is diagnosed without difficulty. Some cases are more apparent than real, in that they represent occult psoriasis. Complete physical examination and history may help make this diagnosis. A work relationship may be present if chronic friction and irritation are discovered in the work process.

Reference

Freeman S: Diagnosis and differential diagnosis. In Adams RM (ed): Occupational Skin Disease, 2nd ed. Philadelphia, WB Saunders, 1990, p 207.

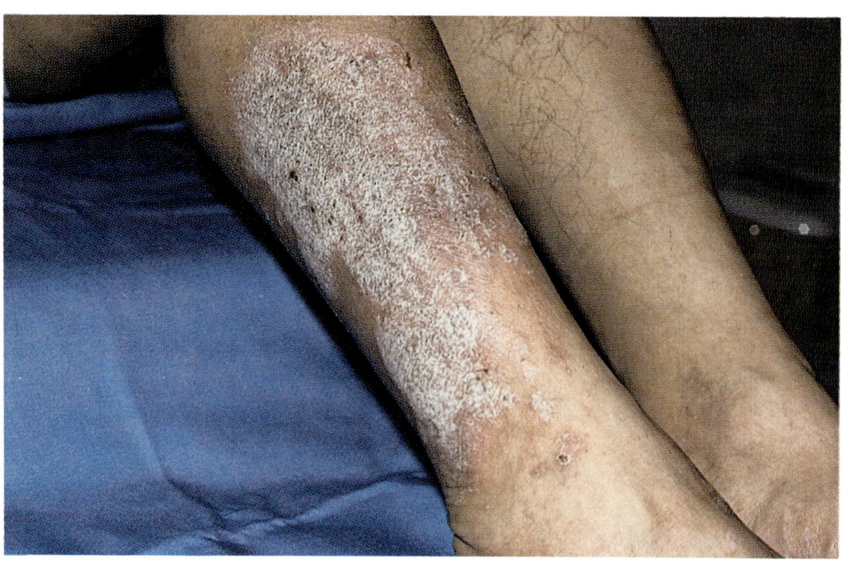

LICHEN SIMPLEX CHRONICUS

SELF-EXCORIATION OF THE FACE

HISTORY

A 43-year-old woman consulted a physician for painful lesions on the forehead and cheeks of several years' duration. Healing is slow and new areas appear without obvious cause. Scarring results in nearly every instance. Patch testing was not done. Biopsy showed a subacute ulcer.

RESOLUTION

From the geometric appearance of each lesion a diagnosis of self-inflicted ulcerations was made. The patient denied manipulating these areas, but the ulcerations appeared to have been caused by an instrument in addition to her fingernails. On further questioning, she stated she had consulted several other physicians and complained that they had each told her to stop manipulating her skin.

CLINICAL COMMENTS

Self-inflicted wounds of the skin are difficult to treat. When patients admit to traumatizing the areas, they usually claim it necessary either to relieve itching or remove "something" (such as a worm) from the skin. Psychiatric referral is usually required, but psychiatric treatment is infrequently effective.

References

Arnold HL, Odom RB, James WD: Andrews' Diseases of the Skin, 8th ed. Philadelphia, WB Saunders, 1990, pp 63–64.

Lyell A: Cutaneous artifactual disease. J Am Acad Dermatol 1:391, 1979.

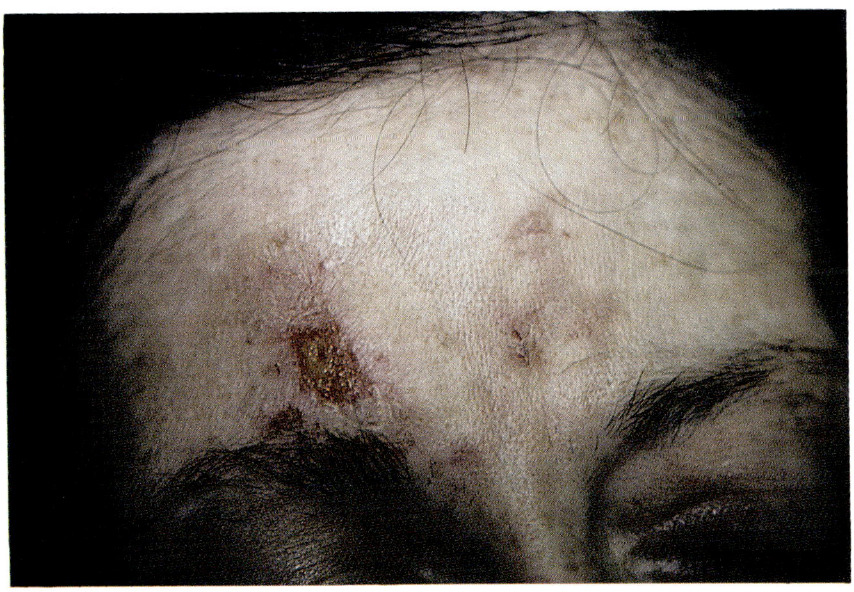

SELF-EXCORIATION OF THE FACE

XEROSIS

HISTORY

A 48-year-old woman with a previous history of atopic dermatitis and asthma developed highly pruritic, sharply demarcated, round and oval lesions on her legs, thighs, abdomen, and arms. The history revealed excessive bathing, using a detergent-type liquid soap and brush. Results of patch testing were negative to a standard series of allergens.

RESOLUTION

Topical medications, over-the-counter emollients, and a decrease in bathing frequency (and duration) are usually sufficient to ameliorate the symptoms. Humidifiers in the bedroom and living room are also helpful, especially in winter.

CLINICAL COMMENTS

Xerosis is common among atopic patients and becomes especially severe as they grow older. A nummular pattern is often seen. Excessive, prolonged showering and bathing are common, and from the history an atopic personal or family background may be elicited.

References

Arnold HL, Odom RB, James WD: Andrews' Diseases of the Skin, 8th ed. Philadelphia, WB Saunders, 1990, p 81.

Shelley WB, Shelley ED: Xerosis. In Advanced Dermatologic Therapy. Philadelphia, WB Saunders, 1987, pp 542–543.

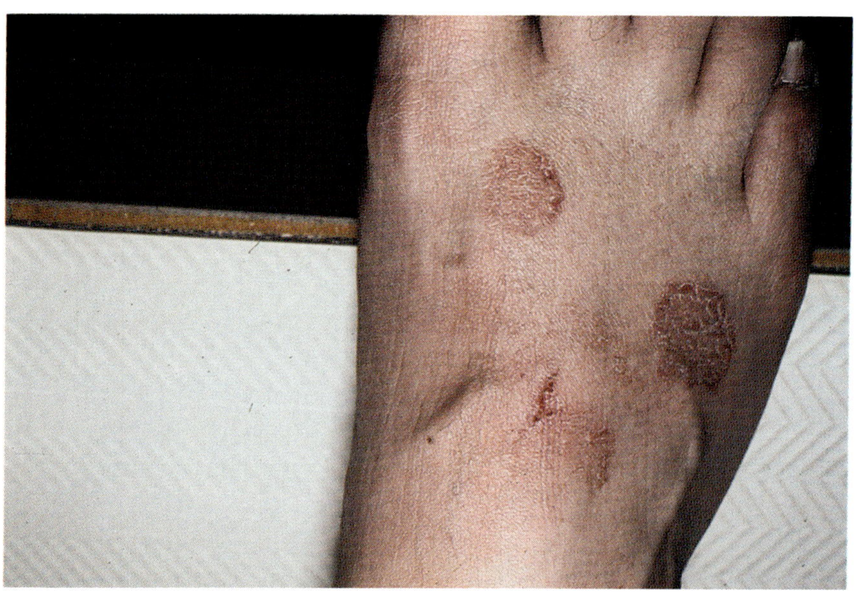

Courtesy of Frances J. Storrs, M.D.

XEROSIS

BOWEN'S DISEASE

HISTORY

A small, dry, scaling lesion at the base of the left index finger has slowly increased in size over several years. In spite of the absence of itching, the 35-year-old patient was thought to have contact dermatitis and was referred for patch testing. Biopsy showed intraepidermal squamous cell carcinoma (Bowen's disease).

RESOLUTION

Excision with primary closure was effective. No other lesions were found. A history of oral arsenical ingestion (Gay's solution) for childhood asthma was elicited.

CLINICAL COMMENTS

Bowen's disease may resemble contact dermatitis, although there is no pruritus or vesiculation. The lesions are sharply demarcated. Although its relationship to oral arsenic is still controversial and in many cases cannot be documented, in this case there seemed to be some evidence to support this contention.

References

Callen J, Headington J: Bowen's and non-Bowen's squamous intraepidermal neoplasia of the skin. Arch Dermatol 116:422–426, 1980.

Epstein E: Association of Bowen's disease with visceral cancer. Arch Dermatol 82:349–351, 1960.

Miki Y, Kawatsu T, Matsuda K, et al: Cutaneous and pulmonary cancers associated with Bowen's disease. J Am Acad Dermatol 6:26–31, 1982.

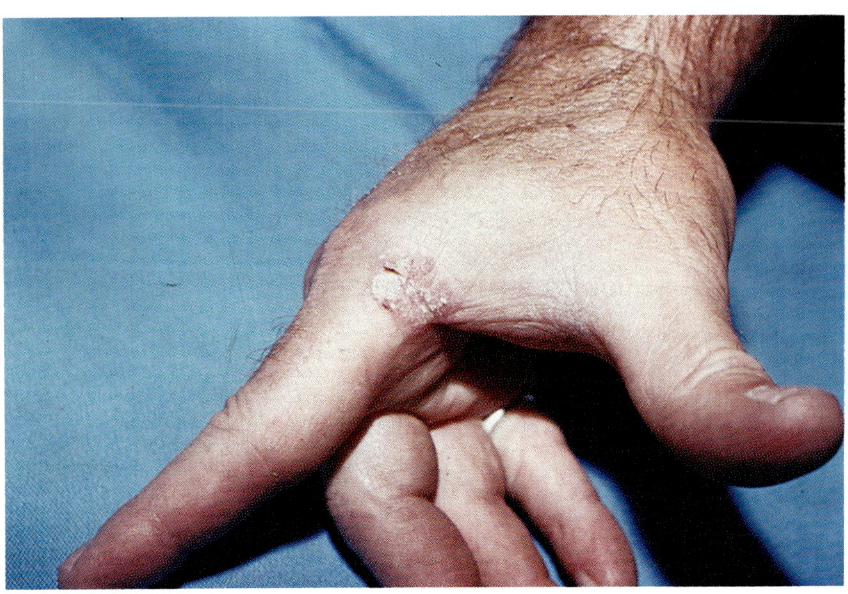

BOWEN'S DISEASE

SECONDARY SYPHILIS

HISTORY

A 23-year-old homosexual man presented with a widespread macular, slightly scaling eruption on the trunk, arms, legs, and face, with recently developing lesions on the palms. These were slightly tender on pressure. Generalized lymphadenopathy was present and the patient felt "under par." Serologic tests for syphilis were strongly positive, and a history of a penile ulcer 3 weeks previously was elicited.

RESOLUTION

A single intramuscular injection of 2.4 million units of penicillin G benzathine or eight daily intramuscular injections of 600,000 units of penicillin G procaine usually suffice, except in HIV infections.

CLINICAL COMMENTS

Although syphilis is still considered "the great imitator," it is unlikely today that secondary syphilis would be confused with contact dermatitis. However, when the trunk is primarily involved and pruritus is slight, clothing dermatitis might be considered. Careful examination of the mucous membranes, palms, and soles should aid in the diagnosis, however.

Reference

Arnold HL, Odom RB, James WD: Andrews' Diseases of the Skin. Philadelphia, WB Saunders, 1990, pp 405–429.

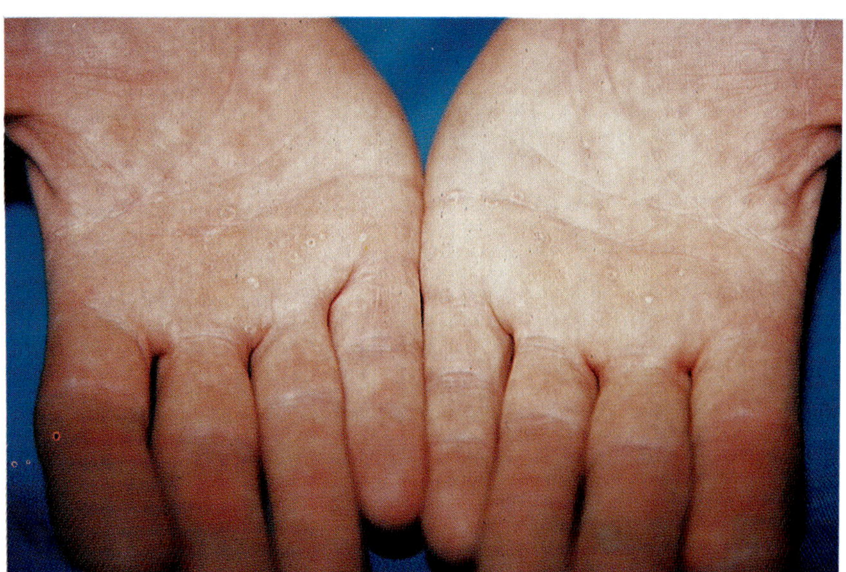

SECONDARY SYPHILIS

ATOPIC DERMATITIS

HISTORY

This man presented with a long history of dermatitis of the face and the antecubital fossae. He was thought to have contact dermatitis, but results of patch testing to common allergens were negative.

RESOLUTION

The dermatitis responded only partially to a topical corticosteroid preparation.

CLINICAL COMMENTS

Dermatitis in patients with atopic dermatitis can mimic contact dermatitis. Patients with long-standing and poorly controlled atopic dermatitis should be patch tested to rule out the possibility of secondary contact dermatitis. However, many atopic patients tend to be hyporeactive to contact allergens.

Reference

Solomon LM: Atopic dermatitis. In Moschella SL, Hurley HJ: Dermatology, 2nd ed. Philadelphia, WB Saunders, 1985, pp 334–353.

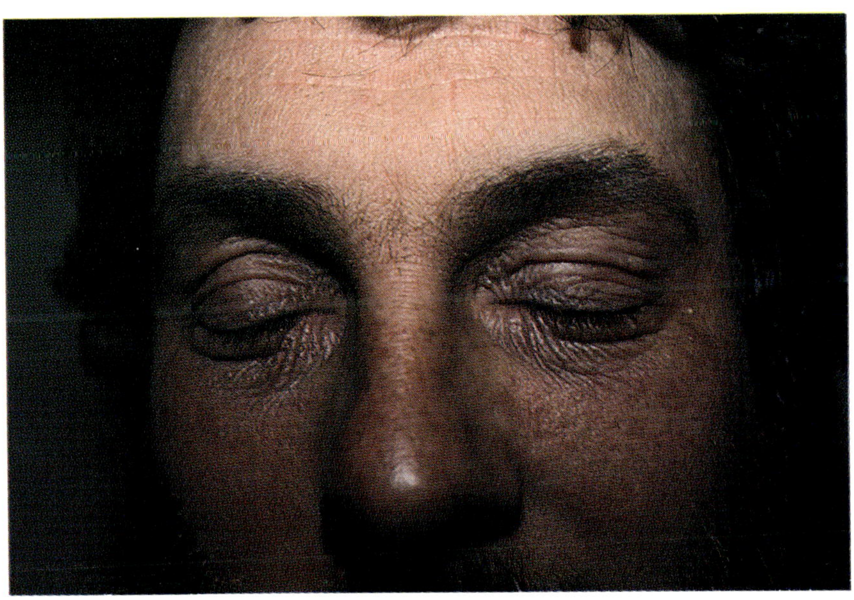

ATOPIC DERMATITIS

SEBORRHEIC DERMATITIS

HISTORY

A patient presented with an erythematous eruption over the nose and cheek area that was well demarcated. Itching was minimal. There also was scaling in the ears and scalp.

RESOLUTION

The seborrheic dermatitis cleared readily with application of ketoconazole cream to the face and the use of selenium sulfide shampoo.

CLINICAL COMMENTS

Seborrheic dermatitis can sometimes be confused with contact dermatitis, especially cosmetic dermatitis on the face. Seborrheic dermatitis usually is nonpruritic, whereas contact dermatitis nearly always is pruritic. However, itching on the scalp and in the ear can be quite intense. Ketoconazole is specific for the pathogenic yeast *Pityrosporum ovale*, which causes seborrheic dermatitis.

Reference

Shelley WB, Shelley D: Advanced Dermatologic Therapy. Philadelphia, WB Saunders, 1987, pp 471–476.

ROSACEA

HISTORY

This middle-aged woman has been developing erythematous papules and some pustules on the nose and cheeks for the last several years. She believed she was allergic to something because several of her moisturizers seemed to make the condition worse.

RESOLUTION

The rosacea was treated with tetracycline and completely resolved.

CLINICAL COMMENTS

Rosacea sometimes can be confused with contact dermatitis. However, patients with rosacea almost never cite itching as a prominent complaint. Iatrogenic rosacea commonly results from the use of potent topical corticoids on the face.

Reference

Shelley WB, Shelley D: Advanced Dermatologic Therapy. Philadelphia. WB Saunders, 1987, pp 446–451.

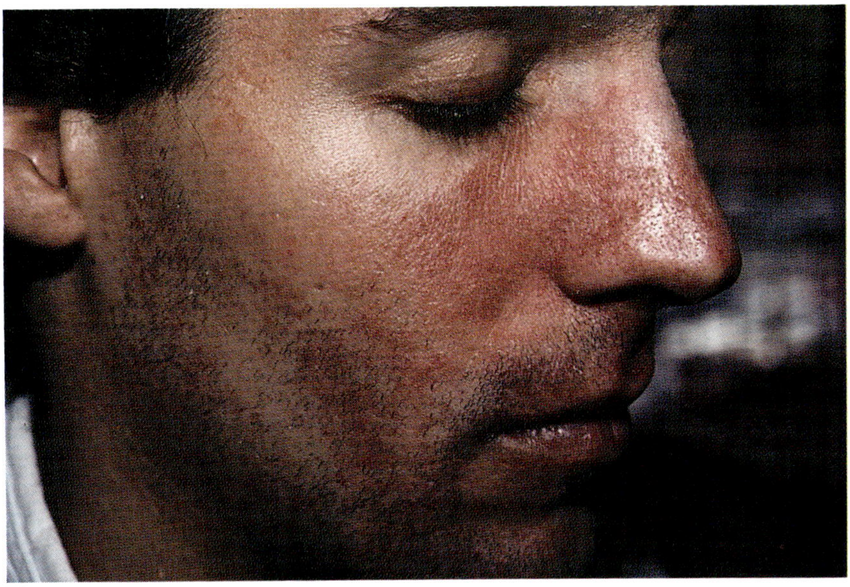

SEBORRHEIC DERMATITIS

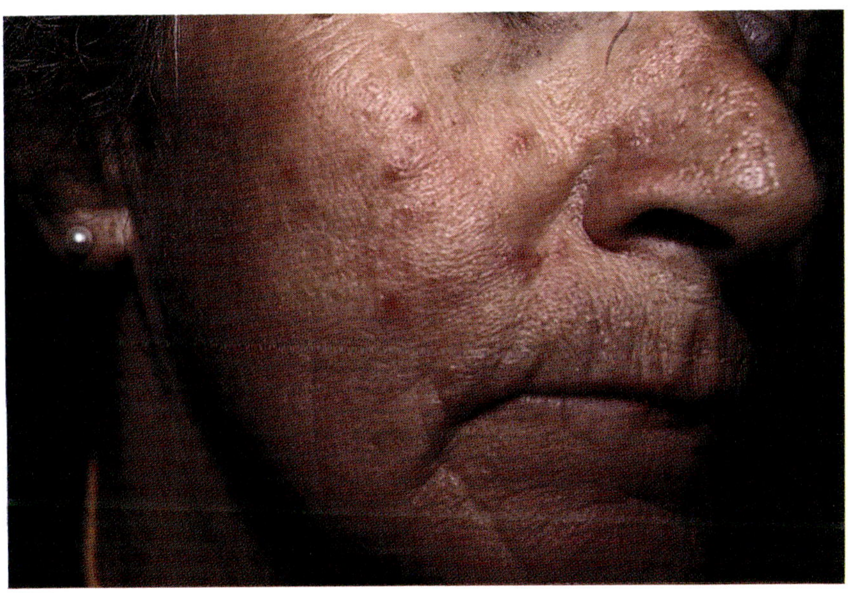

ROSACEA

HERPES ZOSTER

HISTORY

This man developed a pruritic, painful eruption on the right side of the forehead, nose, and scalp. He had been in the woods and thought he had developed poison oak.

RESOLUTION

The distribution and pain suggested zoster. A positive Tzanck preparation showing giant cells confirmed the diagnosis.

CLINICAL COMMENTS

Vesicles on an erythematous base in a dermatomal distribution is a pattern fairly typical of zoster. However, it may sometimes be confused with acute contact dermatitis, especially a weed dermatitis such as poison ivy or oak. Moderate to severe zoster is generally treated with systemic corticosteroids and/or acyclovir.

Reference

Shelley WB, Shelley D: Advanced Dermatologic Therapy. Philadelphia, WB Saunders, 1987, pp 242–248.

HERPES SIMPLEX

HISTORY

This young man went skiing and developed dermatitis on the right side of his cheek. He related that in the past sunlight exposure seemed to trigger this type of eruption.

RESOLUTION

A Tzanck preparation showing giant cells supported the diagnosis of herpes simplex. He responded readily to oral acyclovir. He was advised to apply a broad spectrum sunblock in the future.

CLINICAL COMMENTS

Grouped vesicles on an erythematous base can sometimes be mistaken for acute contact dermatitis. A careful history and a Tzanck preparation are helpful in distinguishing herpes simplex. Recurrent herpes simplex tends to favor the identical site each time. Sunlight commonly precipitates herpes simplex. A culture is required to confirm the diagnosis.

Reference

Shelley WB, Shelley D: Advanced Dermatologic Therapy. Philadelphia, WB Saunders, 1987, pp 235–241.

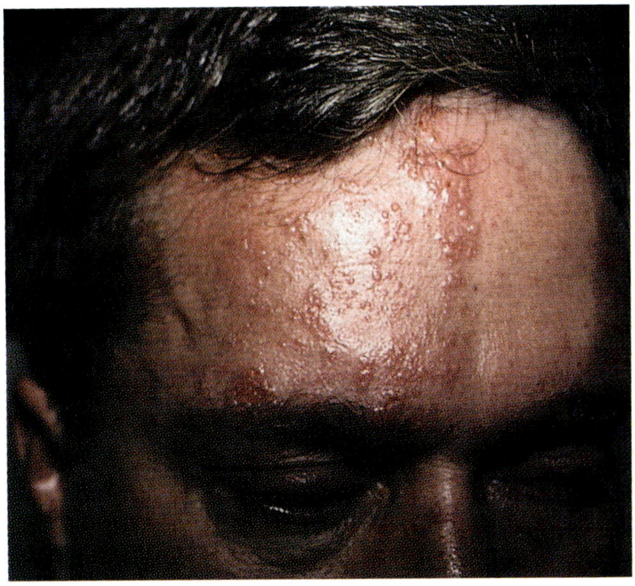

HERPES ZOSTER

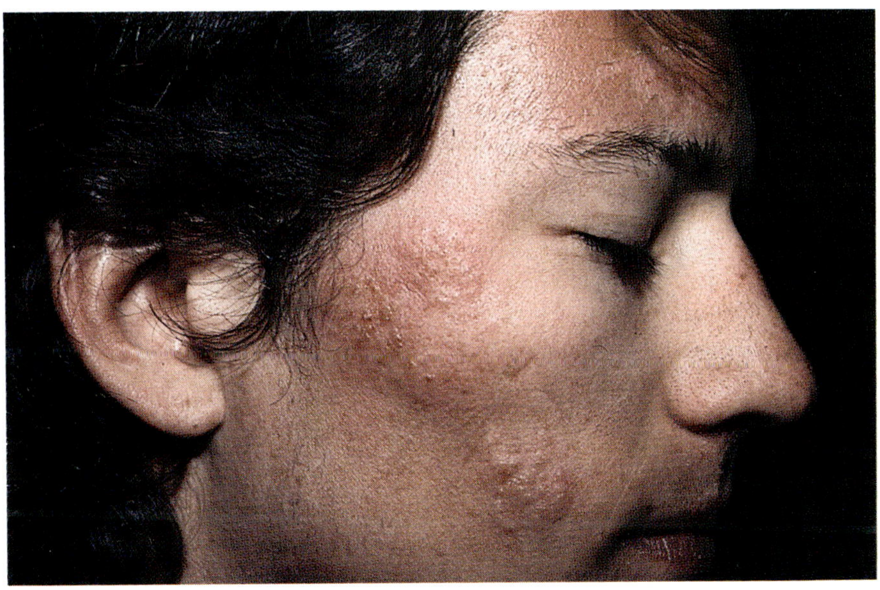

HERPES SIMPLEX

TINEA MANUUM

HISTORY

This patient presented with an acute eruption on the back of the left hand that was very pruritic and sharply demarcated.

RESOLUTION

A potassium hydroxide (KOH) preparation from the peripheral scale revealed the presence of multiple hyphae. Griseofulvin taken orally and a topical antifungal agent completely resolved the eruption.

CLINICAL COMMENTS

Acute tinea infections can sometimes be confused with acute contact dermatitis. The presence of a sharp, well-demarcated, scaling border strongly suggests the diagnosis. Tinea usually occurs on the feet, but it may occur on the hands, face, and elsewhere.

Reference

Shelley WB, Shelley D: Advanced Dermatologic Therapy. Philadelphia, WB Saunders, 1987, pp 485–489.

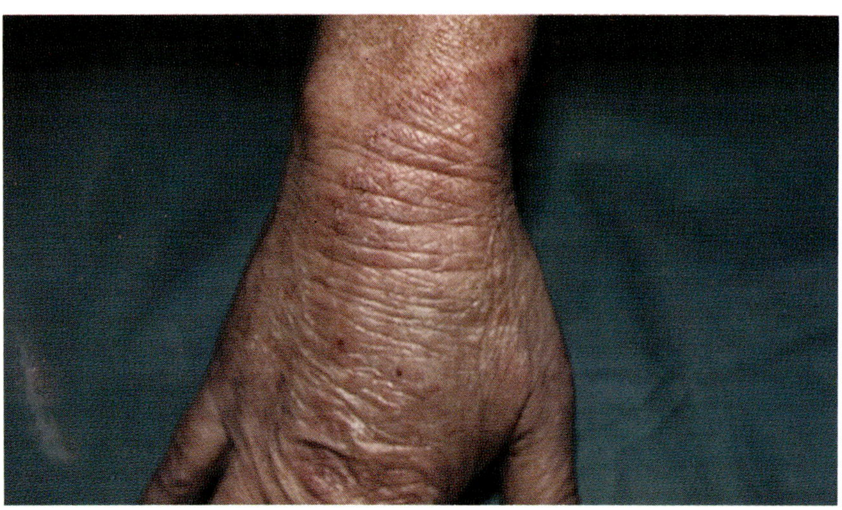

TINEA MANUUM

PERIORAL DERMATITIS

HISTORY

This young woman presented with a recurring eruption around the mouth extending to the nasolabial areas. Mild pruritus was present; the patient suspected a cosmetic allergy due to a certain moisturizer.

RESOLUTION

Diagnosis of perioral dermatitis was made and the patient treated with oral tetracycline and Sulfacet R. Resolution required about 1 month.

CLINICAL COMMENTS

Perioral dermatitis can sometimes be confused with contact dermatitis due to cosmetics. Its etiology is unknown, but the use of potent topical steroids and moisturizing products is a likely etiologic factor. It is important to discontinue application of fluorinated corticosteroids and comedogenic moisturizers and other oil-containing cosmetics. These measures together with tetracycline usually result in resolution.

References

Bendl BJ: Perioral dermatitis: Etiology and treatment. Cutis 17:903–908, 1976.
Fritsch P, Pichler E, Linser I: Periorale dermatitis. Hautarzt 40:475–479, 1989.
Wilkinson DS, Kirton U, Wilkinson JD: Perioral dermatitis: A 12-year review. Br J Dermatol 101(3):245–257, 1979.

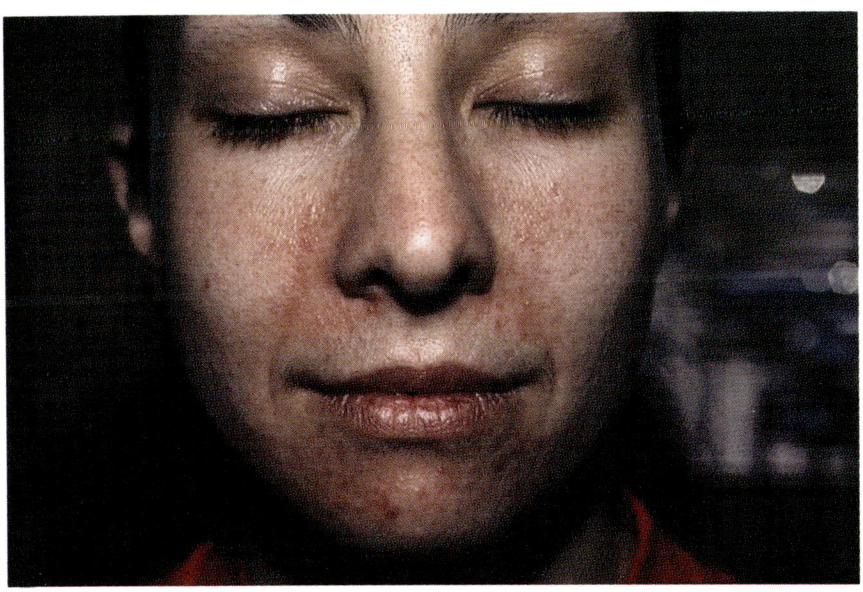

PERIORAL DERMATITIS

POLYMORPHOUS LIGHT ERUPTION

HISTORY

A 14-year-old boy experienced recurring eruptions on the face, arms, and trunk 3 to 4 days following sunlight exposure. He had mild pruritus, vesiculation, and telangiectasis. Contact allergy to a sunscreen was suspected; patch testing and photo patch testing was negative, however. Phototesting with small increments of Ultraviolet B (UVB) over several days duplicated the reaction, which on biopsy strongly suggested a diagnosis of polymorphous light eruption.

RESOLUTION

Treatment is chiefly symptomatic. Psoralen and ultraviolet A phototherapy (PUVA) has been found helpful in some cases, and antimalarial drugs may be useful in severe cases.

CLINICAL COMMENTS

When the eruption is eczematous and limited to the face or hands, a diagnosis of contact dermatitis could be confused, especially allergic contact dermatitis to a cosmetic.

References

Arnold HL, Odom RB, James WD: Andrews' Diseases of the Skin. Philadelphia, WB Saunders, 1990, pp 39–40.

Epstein JH: Polymorphous light eruption. J Am Acad Dermatol 3:329, 1980.

Galosi A, Holzle E, Plewig G, et al: PUVA therapy in persistent light reaction. Hautarzt 33:551–557, 1982.

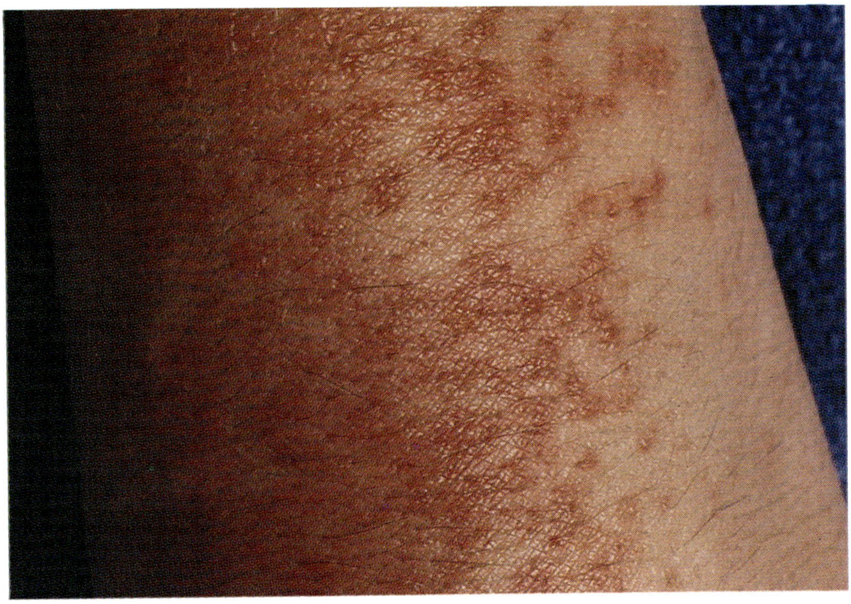

Courtesy of Vincent A. De Leo, M.D.

POLYMORPHOUS LIGHT ERUPTION

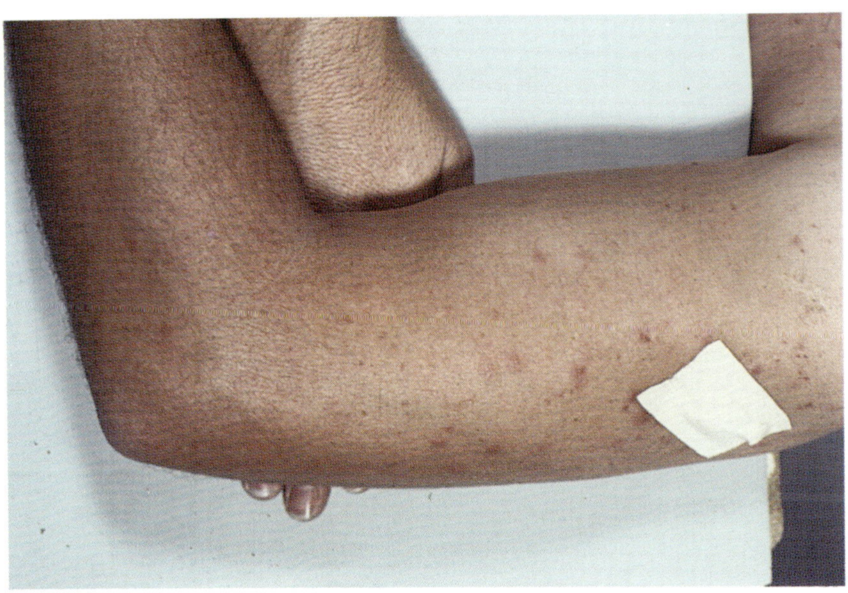

Courtesy of Vincent A. De Leo, M.D.

POLYMORPHOUS LIGHT ERUPTION

LYME DISEASE

HISTORY

Several days after walking in the woods this woman noticed this erythematous and slightly pruritic area on her left trunk. It rapidly enlarged. She remembered seeing deer grazing in the area but could not recall having been bitten by a tick.

RESOLUTION

A diagnosis of erythema chronicum migrans associated with Lyme disease was made. She was treated with 100 mg of minocycline twice a day for 21 days. There was rapid resolution of the dermatitis.

CLINICAL ASPECTS

Erythema chronicum migrans (ECM) occurs in a majority of patients who develop Lyme borreliosis. ECM can be confused with hives, contact dermatitis, or tinea infection. The lesion begins as a small papule following a tick bite. Characteristically, the lesion evolves and enlarges daily, reaching up to 10 to 12 cm in diameter.

A major problem is the lack of reliable immunologic criteria for diagnosis. The preferred treatment of early stage Lyme disease is 300 mg of doxycycline or minocycline for three weeks. The alternative is 100 to 500 mg of amoxicillin three times a day for 21 days plus 500 mg of probenecid three times a day. Herxheimer reactions have been reported to occur.

Reference

Luft BJ, Gorevic PD, Halperin JJ, et al: A perspective on the treatment of Lyme borreliosis. Rev Infect Dis 11(Suppl 6):S1518–S1525, 1989.

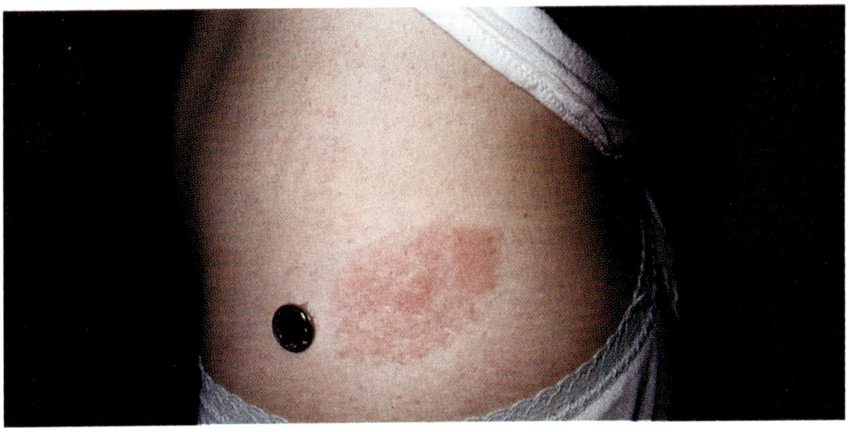

Courtesy of Stephen Luger, M.D.

LYME DISEASE

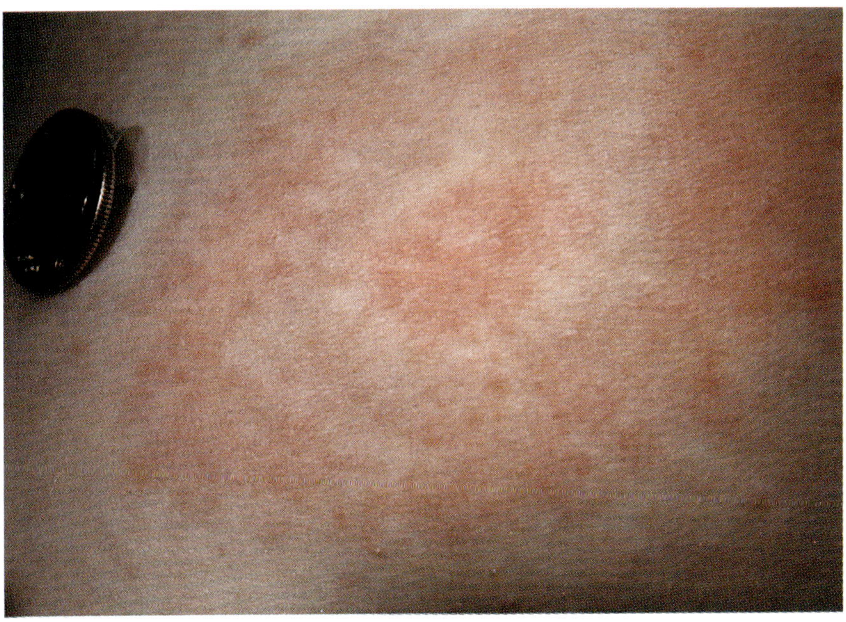

Courtesy of Stephen Luger, M.D.

LYME DISEASE

Section XIV

Systemic Contact Dermatitis

ORALLY ELICITED ALLERGIC CONTACT DERMATITIS (SYSTEMIC CONTACT TYPE DERMATITIS)

Cashew Nut

HISTORY

This patient worked in a cashew nut processing plant. She took home the roasted cashew nuts and consumed a considerable number on the weekend. Dermatitis developed approximately 36 hours later.

RESOLUTION

The eruption required systemic corticosteroid therapy but cleared completely. No further exacerbations occurred after the patient made the diagnosis and discussed it with her dermatologist.

CLINICAL COMMENTS

A diagnosis of allergic "contact" dermatitis from oral ingestion is rarely made, presumably because the condition remains unrecognized by physicians in a majority of cases. Occasionally patients themselves suggest the diagnosis.

Confirmation is made by the finding of a positive patch test to the substance and reproducing the dermatitis by oral ingestion. The risks of oral challenge are minimal, especially if small doses are administered. Although rarely performed by physicians, such provocative tests are important to avoid recurrent episodes of this often disabling dermatitis.

Reference

Veien N, Menné T, Maibach H: Systemically induced allergic contact dermatitis. In Menné T, Maibach H (eds.): Exogenous Dermatoses: Environmental Dermatitis. Boca Raton, FL, CRC Press, 1990, pp 267–282.

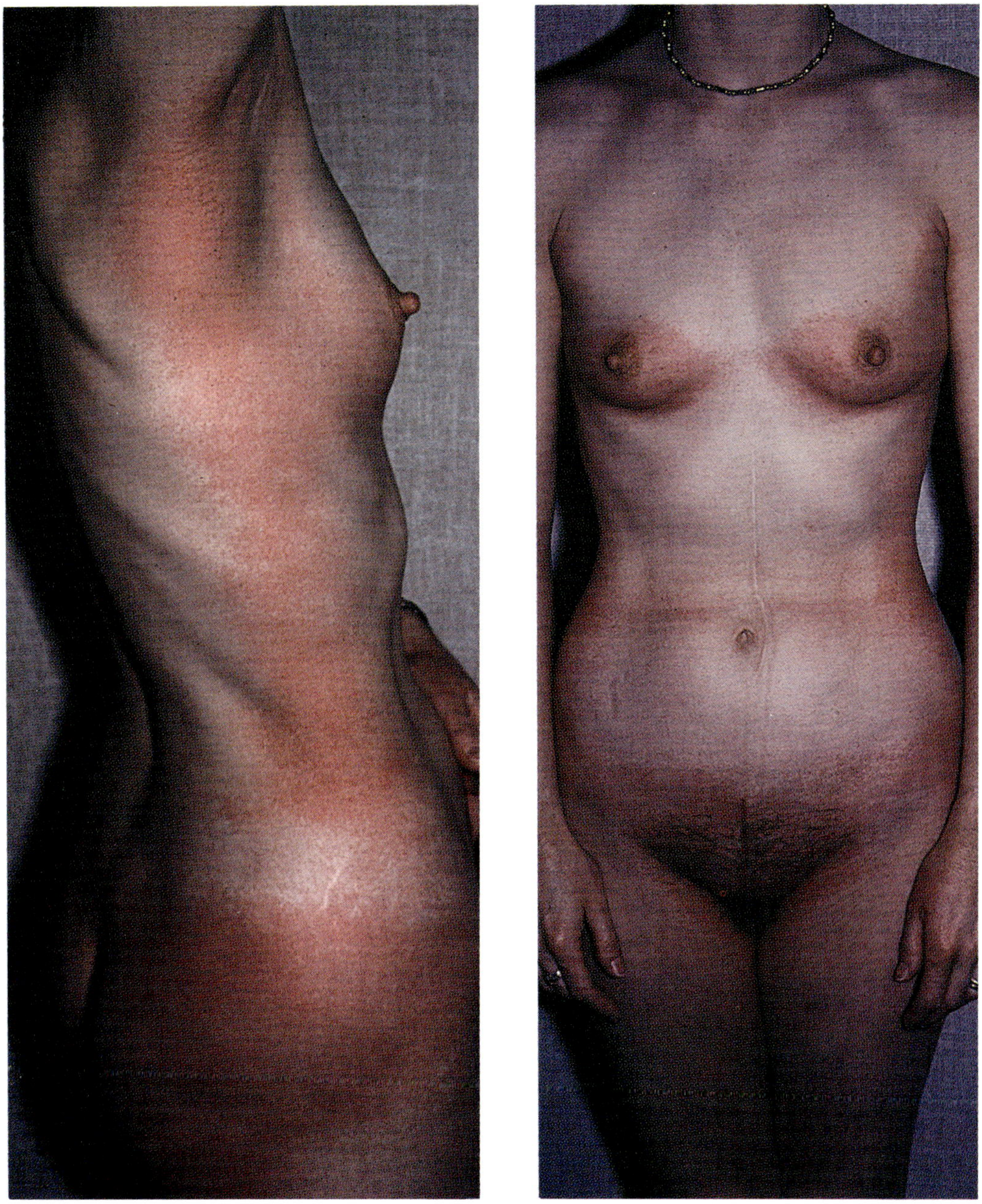

Courtesy of Alan Binnick, M.D.

SYSTEMIC ALLERGIC CONTACT DERMATITIS FROM INGESTION

ORALLY ELICITED ALLERGIC CONTACT DERMATITIS (SYSTEMIC CONTACT DERMATITIS)

Phenergan

HISTORY

A 57-year-old woman developed a severe facial dermatitis following use of promethazine cream (Phenergan), prescribed for her by a physician in Madagascar. Topical treatment and avoidance of further promethazine cream resulted in prompt clearing. Patch testing to the cream was strongly positive. One year later, when back in the United States, she was given oral promethazine by her physician for an upper respiratory infection. Within 18 hours she developed a generalized, erythematous, highly pruritic eruption requiring hospitalization.

RESOLUTION

The eruption was consistent with exfoliative dermatitis but resolved completely following appropriate treatment. The patient was provided with a list of medications related to promethazine, and she was advised to keep the list readily available in the future.

CLINICAL COMMENTS

So-called "systemic contact dermatitis" is infrequently diagnosed, usually resulting from oral or parenteral administration of a substance that previously has induced contact allergic sensitization. The sulfonamides and their derivatives are the frequent causes.

References

Epstein S: Allergic photocontact dermatitis from promethazine (Phenergan). Arch Dermatol Syph 81:175, 1960.

Fisher AA: Systemic contact-type dermatitis. In Fisher AA: Contact Dermatitis, 3rd ed. Philadelphia, Lea & Febiger, 1986, pp 119–130.

Menne T, Veien N, Maibach H: Systemic contact-type dermatitis due to drugs. Semin Dermatol 8:144–148, 1989.

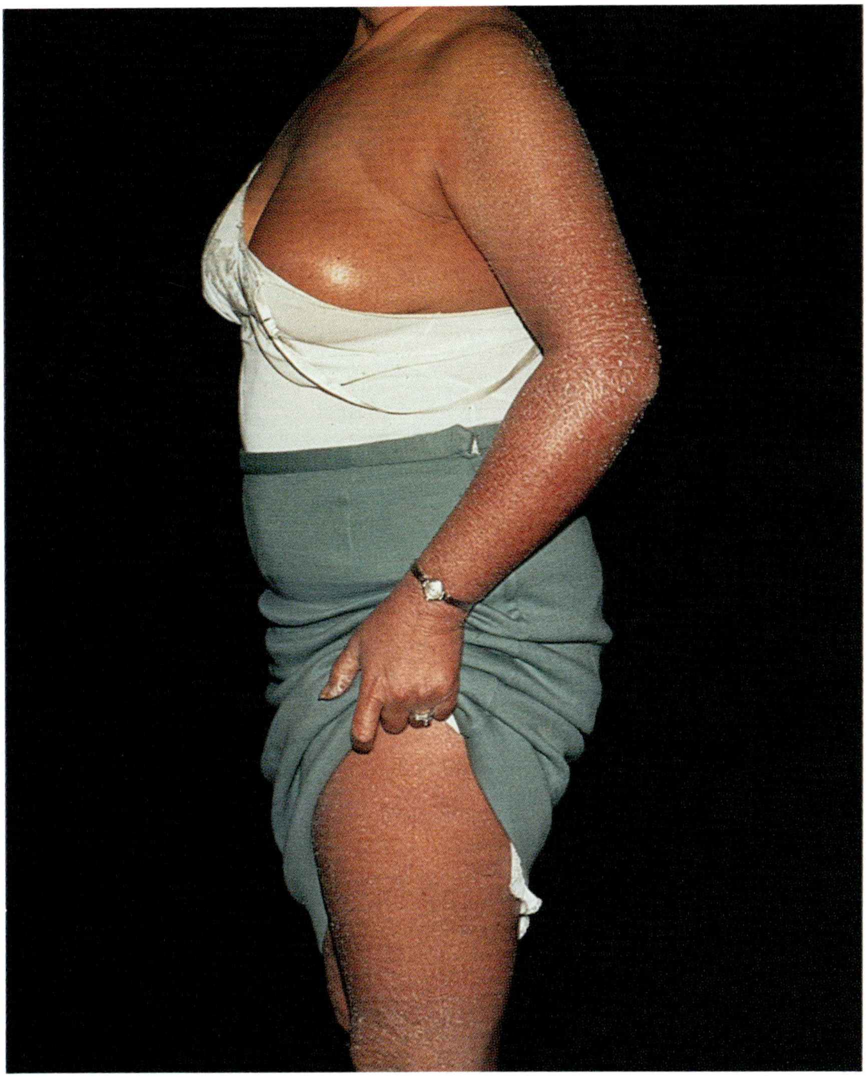

SYSTEMIC CONTACT DERMATITIS

BABOON SYNDROME

HISTORY

This patient had normal skin until recent oral administration of a sulfonamide. Within approximately 48 hours after consuming a normal dose, the patient noted a severe dermatitis of the abdomen, buttocks, and body folds.

RESOLUTION

On the basis of history and morphology, a diagnosis of drug reaction of the "baboon syndrome" type was made, and the drug was discontinued.

CLINICAL COMMENTS

Baboon syndrome is one of the many variants of drug eruptions; what is so unusual is the striking predilection for the anatomic sites noted here. The name was derived by the late Dr. Niels Hjorth because of similarity of the reaction to those seen during the estrus cycle in the baboon.

Some patients with baboon syndrome may have delayed hypersensitivity because they show positive patch test results to the material.

Provocative drug challenges, such as that utilized by Kauppinen, for many drugs (with a remarkable safety record) have not been systematically applied to the baboon syndrome variant of drug reaction.

References

Anderson KE, Hjorth N, Menne T: The baboon syndrome: Systemically induced allergic contact dermatitis. Contact Dermatitis 10:97–100, 1984.

Kauppinen K, Alanko K: Oral provocation, uses. Semin Derm 8:187–191, 1989.

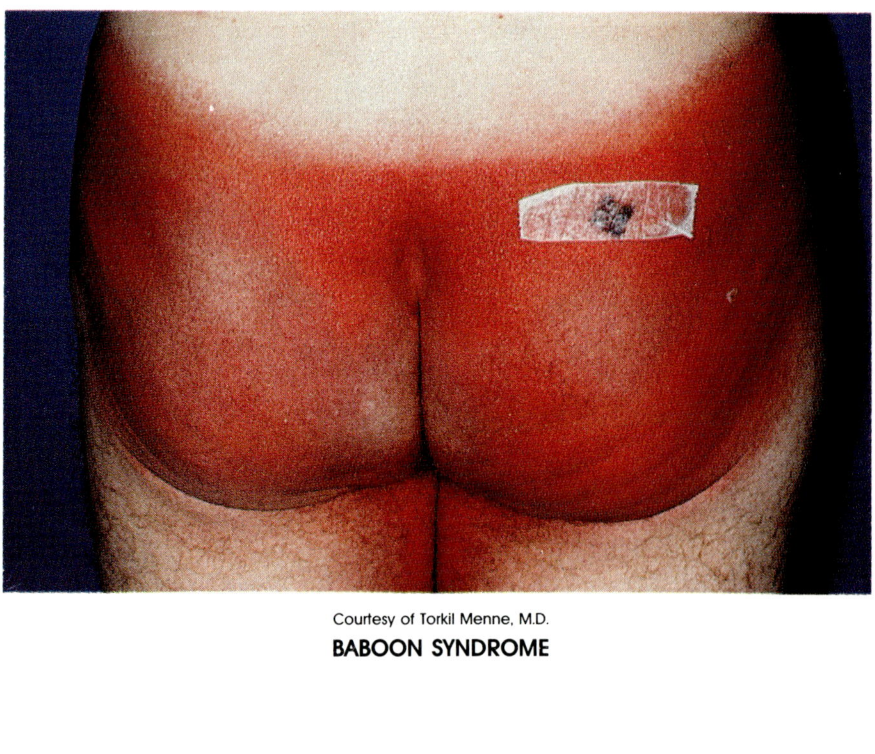

Courtesy of Torkil Menne, M.D.

BABOON SYNDROME

Section XV

Spot Tests

DIMETHYLGLYOXIME SPOT TEST FOR NICKEL

This useful test kit for the presence of nickel on jewelry, buttons, and other metal objects contains 1% dimethylglyoxime (DMG) in alcohol and 10% ammonium hydroxide solution. Developed for dermatologic use by Alexander A. Fisher, the test is now widely used by dermatologists. The directions are as follows: Apply one or two drops of the DMG solution (container A) to the part to be tested and add one or two drops of the ammonium hydroxide solution (container B); mix with a Q-tip or cotton applicator, and observe the color on the cotton. A deep pink color, as demonstrated on the coins in the photograph, indicates the presence of nickel at greater than 5 parts per million (ppm).

The test (Allertest Ni) is available from Allerderm Laboratories, PO Box 931, Mill Valley, CA 94941. Recently available is a kit containing a predosed swab in a single container, available from Hermal-Chemie, PO Box 1228, D-2057 Reinbek/Hamburg, West Germany.

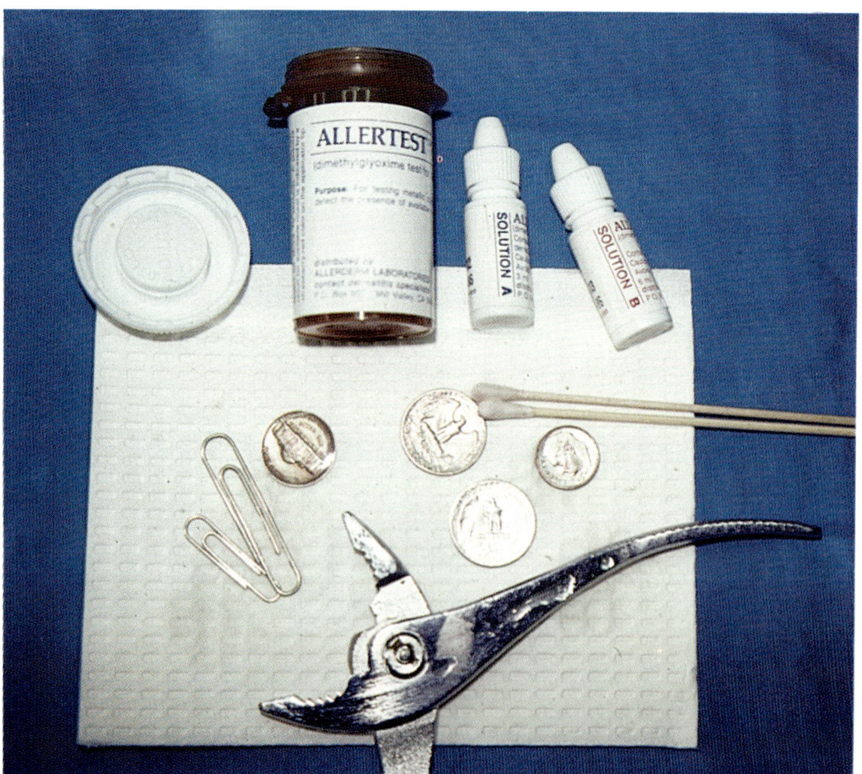

DIMETHYLGLYOXIME SPOT TEST KIT

Section XVI

Urticaria

CONTACT URTICARIA TO CHEESE

HISTORY

This 2-year-old girl developed an urticarial eruption around her mouth immediately after eating cheese, especially when on pizza. The eruption would last several hours. Scratch tests to the cheese were positive.

RESOLUTION

The patient avoided cheese products and had no recurrence.

CLINICAL COMMENTS

Contact urticaria can be either nonimmunologic or immunologic. The nonimmunologic type is the most common and occurs without previous sensitization. Caution should be observed in skin testing since anaphylactoid reactions have been reported in the immunologic type.

Reference

vonKrogh G, Maibach HI: Contact urticaria syndrome. In Moschella SL, Hurley HJ: Dermatology. Philadelphia, WB Saunders, 1985, pp 323–333.

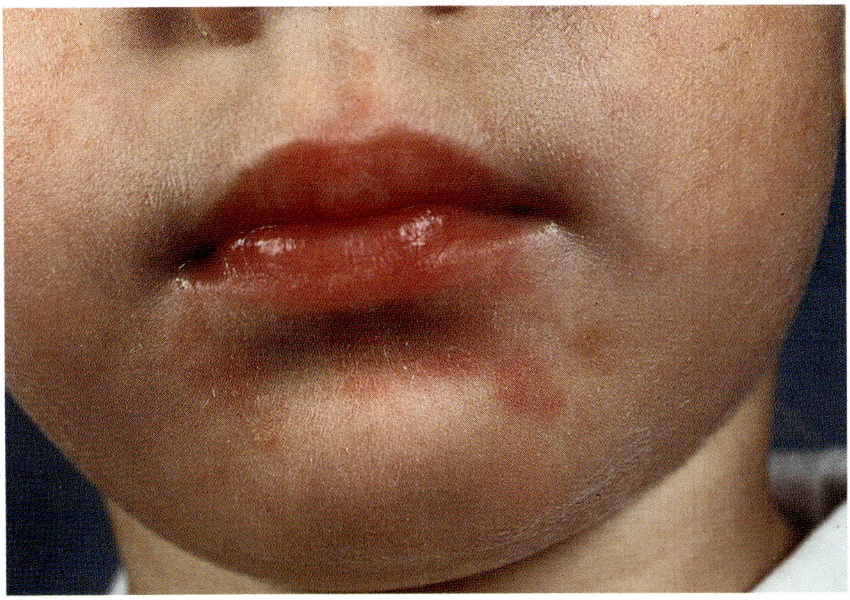

Courtesy of Ronald R. Brancaccio, M.D.

CONTACT URTICARIA FROM CHEESE

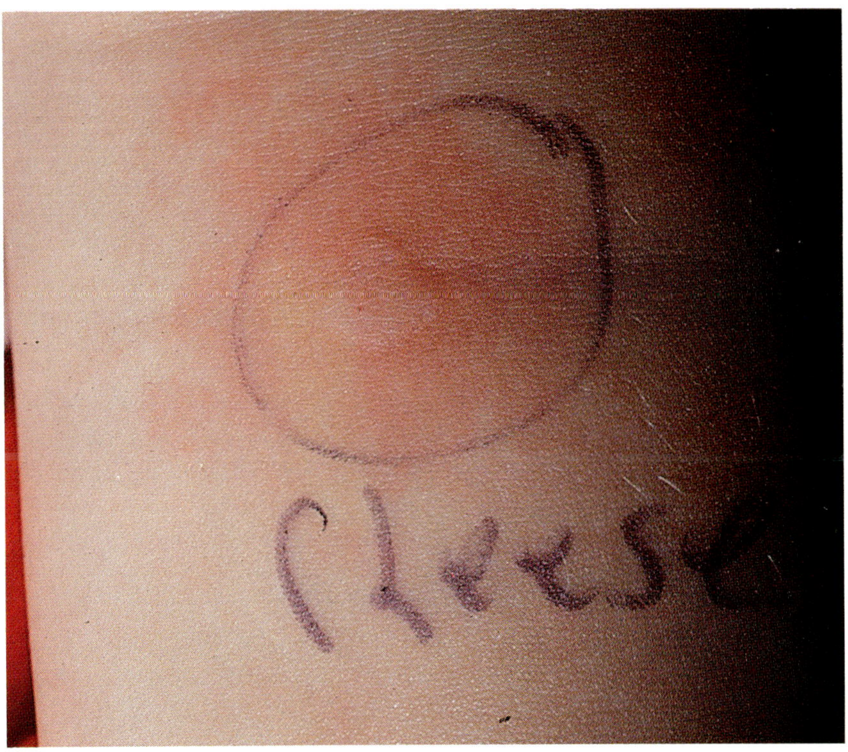

Courtesy of Ronald R. Brancaccio, M.D.

SCRATCH TEST FOR CHEESE

CONTACT URTICARIA TO FRUITS AND VEGETABLES

HISTORY

A young woman developed burning, stinging, itching, and a poorly defined rash on her hands after handling certain fruits and vegetables. Immediate type allergy testing by application of small pieces of these materials to the intact skin on her forehead and forearm revealed the positive reactions shown in the illustration (*A*). *B* demonstrates the reaction to apples, which in this woman, following ingesting, resulted in generalized urticaria.

RESOLUTION

The patient had no further difficulty when she avoided these food products.

CLINICAL COMMENT

Foods may cause allergic and nonallergic contact rashes. Reactions are usually on the hands, but the perioral area may be affected.

References

Hausen BM, Hjorth N: Skin reactions to topical food exposure. Dermatol Clin 2(4):567–578, 1984.

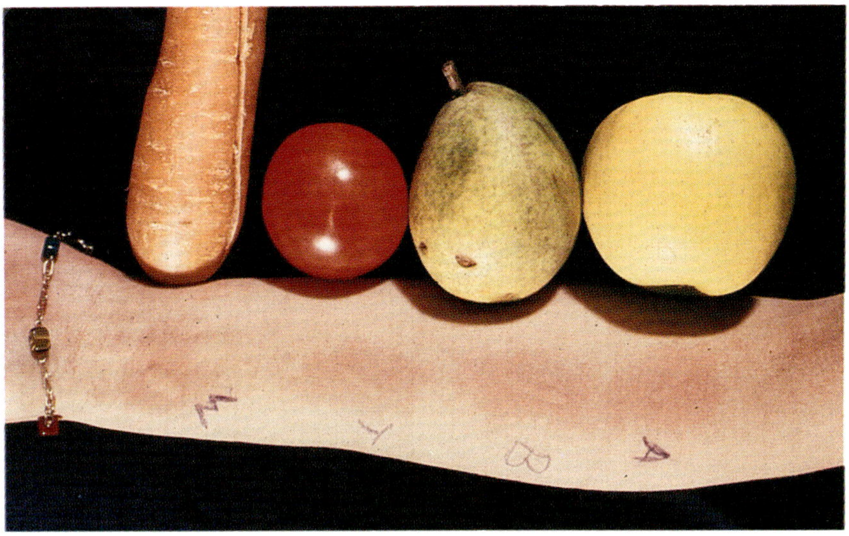

Courtesy of Niels Hjorth, M.D.

CONTACT URTICARIA FROM FRUITS AND VEGETABLES

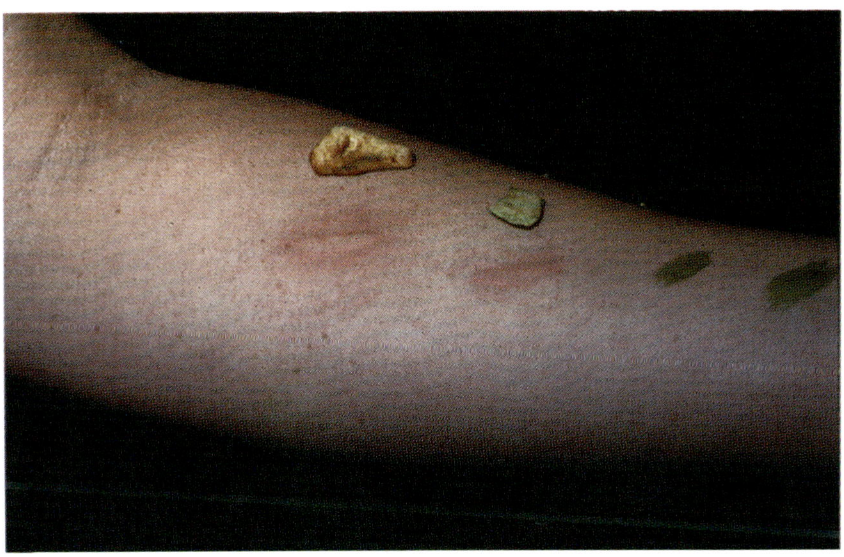

Courtesy of Niels Hjorth, M.D.

CONTACT URTICARIA FROM APPLES

IMMUNOLOGIC CONTACT URTICARIA (ICU)

HISTORY

Photographs *A* and *B* demonstrate erythema and edema. *C* reveals testing on an untreated site: reproduction of the lesion on normal skin. This patient wore latex gloves.

RESOLUTION

ICU usually resolves spontaneously. However, if systemic symptoms are present, such as laryngeal edema, asthma, and anaphylactoid reactions, prompt medical intervention is indicated. Epinephrine, antihistamines, and appropriate supportive therapy are indicated.

CLINICAL COMMENTS

ICU has become a frequently reported phenomenon in recent years. Case reports emphasize its profound medical significance for patients, especially those with ICU to latex gloves. Many of these patients have been misdiagnosed in the past. In almost every case, documentation can be made on the basis of history and a positive provocation test, which consists in either the patient wearing the gloves for 20 to 30 minutes or testing normal skin with a piece of the glove. One must remember that anaphylactoid reactions may occur even with brief exposure; vaginal examination, for example, with a latex glove may induce this reaction in sensitized individuals. Fatal reactions have been documented from barium enema-related latex exposure.

Patients with a history of reactions to latex should notify their physicians of their sensitivity and also keep the information readily available on a bracelet or in their wallet or purse. Most surgeons wear latex gloves during surgery, which may cause disastrous reactions in sensitized patients undergoing surgery.

Reference

Lahti A, Maibach H: Immediate contact reactions. In Menne T, Maibach H (eds.): Exogenous Dermatoses: Environmental Dermatitis. Boca Raton, FL, CRC Press, 1990, pp 21–36.

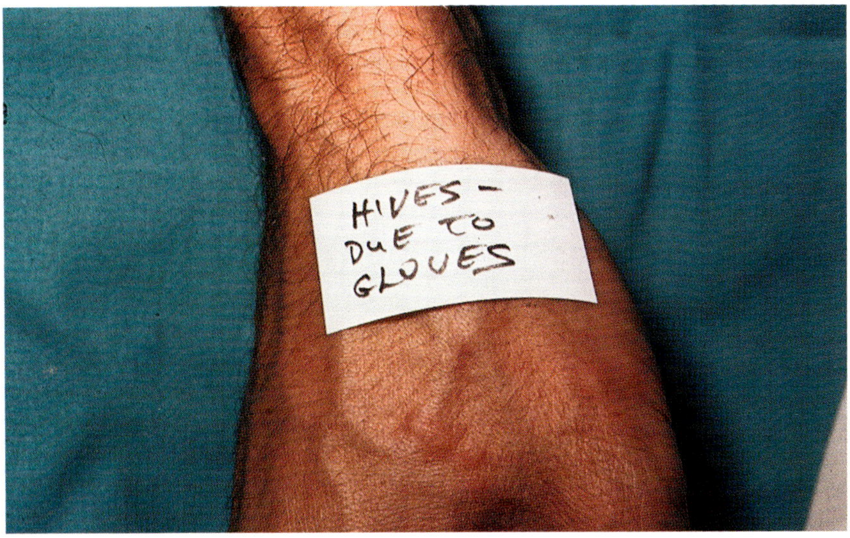

A

Courtesy of James Taylor, M.D.

IMMUNOLOGIC CONTACT URTICARIA

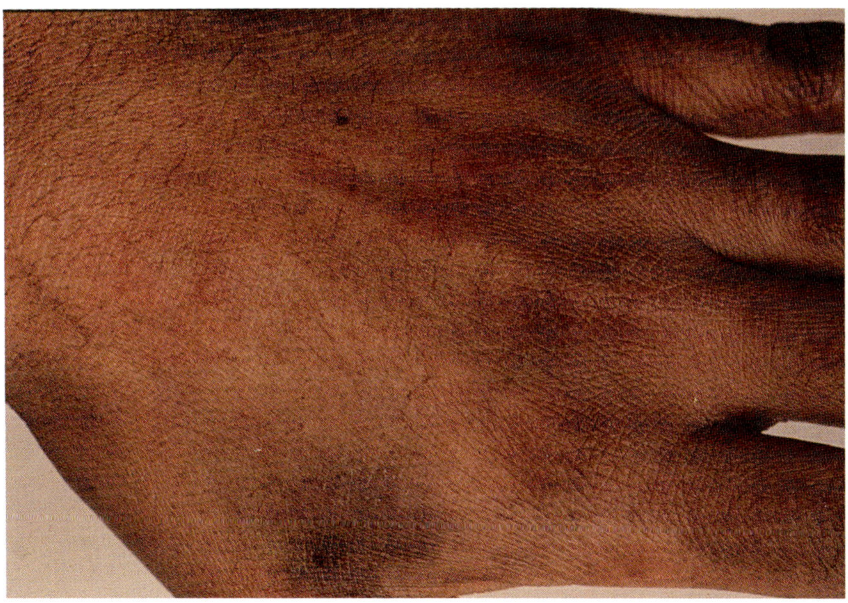

B

Courtesy of James Taylor, M.D.

IMMUNOLOGIC CONTACT URTICARIA

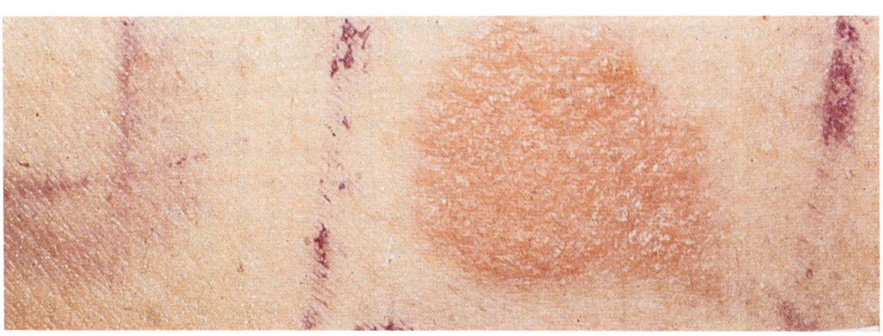

C

Courtesy of James Taylor, M.D.

IMMUNOLOGIC CONTACT URTICARIA TEST SITE (LATEX GLOVE)

CONTACT URTICARIA, NONIMMUNOLOGIC (NICU)

HISTORY

Nonimmunologic contact urticaria in a normal individual is shown. The urticants include benzoic and cinnamic acids.

RESOLUTION

NICU routinely clears on removal of the urticant.

CLINICAL COMMENTS

NICU is very common, but the condition is rarely seen by physicians because the symptoms have usually disappeared by the time the patients seek professional help. Typically, patients relate a history of burning, stinging, and itching and often a transient erythema or perhaps urtication, following application of a product.

Because of its frequency, the condition has been extensively studied. It is typical for a site to react and then remain unreactive for hours or days (tachyphylaxis). In experimental animals, NICU tachyphylaxis may last for up to 2 weeks. Regional variations in reactivity also occur; for example, the face is usually more reactive than the leg. Patients who complain of burning, stinging, and itching should be asked whether they also develop redness and hives, and if so, contact urticaria testing on normal skin is indicated.

Antihistamines may partially inhibit the reaction, and prostaglandin inhibitors are effective in certain nonimmunologic contact urticarial reactions.

References

Maibach H, Johnson H: Contact urticaria syndrome. Arch Dermatol 111:726–730, 1975.

Lahti A, Maibach H: Contact skin allergy. II. Contract urticaria. In Middleton E, Reed C, Ellis F, et al (eds.): Allergy: Principle and Practice, 3rd ed. St Louis, CV Mosby, 1988, pp 1463–1468.

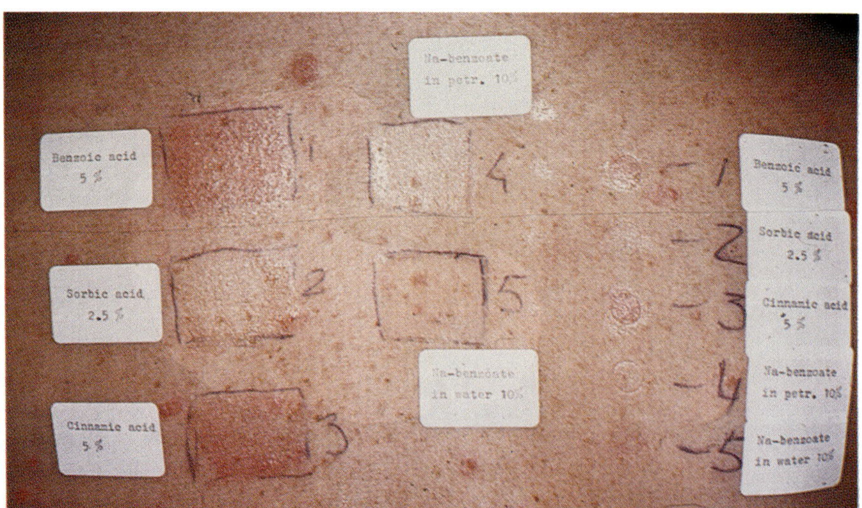

Courtesy of Arto Lahti, M.D.

CONTACT URTICARIA, NONIMMUNOLOGIC

Section XVII

Metals

GOLD ELECTROPLATING

HISTORY

A 21-year-old man had worked in electroplating gold for several months before this pruritic dermatitis appeared in areas where the electroplating solution had splashed onto his arms. His hands were always protected by gloves. Patch testing revealed a strongly positive reaction to 0.5% gold sodium thiosulfate; the reaction persisted for nearly 3 months.

RESOLUTION

Because the patient was an apprentice electroplater, he was not retrained and entered a rehabilitation program for a different type of work. It would have been possible for him to move to another type of electroplating, such as chrome or nickel, probably without recurrence.

CLINICAL COMMENTS

Allergic contact sensitivity to gold is uncommon. Patch testing must be done with gold thiosulfate. Gold chloride is irritating at 1%, and testing with gold leaf is usually negative.

References

Burrows D, Adams RM: Metals. In Adams RM (ed): Occupational Skin Disease, 2nd ed. Philadephia, WB Saunders, 1990, pp 367–369.

Fowler JG: Selection of patch test materials for gold allergy. Contact Dermatitis 17:23–25, 1987.

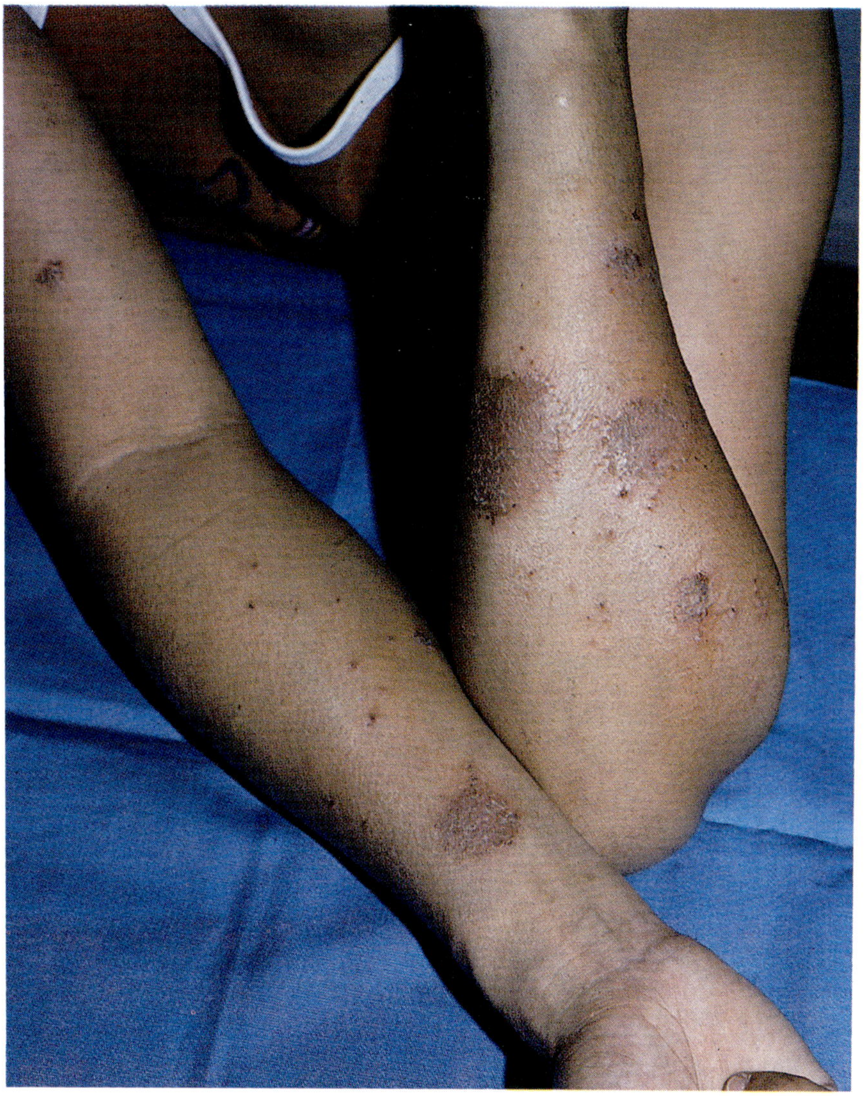

GOLD ELECTROPLATING

Section XVIII

Irritants

ALKALINE SOLVENT

HISTORY

A rookie police officer, wearing cloth gloves, was cleaning his gun with solvent. The solvent spilled and he wiped it up with his gloved hand and continued cleaning for 30 minutes or more. Within about 45 minutes he noted burning of the skin of his palm, and by that evening he noticed blistering. Patch testing was not done.

RESOLUTION

The blisters required 1 week to resolve with considerable desquamation. Scarring did not result. Although the palm was tender for several weeks, eventually complete healing resulted.

CLINICAL COMMENTS

Irritant dermatitis commonly occurs from solvents, especially when they are held against the skin for several hours as a compress. The lesion resembles a burn, which at times may be deep, leaving scarring.

Reference

Shmunes E: Solvents and plasticizers. In Adams RM (ed): Occupational Skin Disease, 2nd ed. Philadelphia, WB Saunders, 1990, pp 439–462.

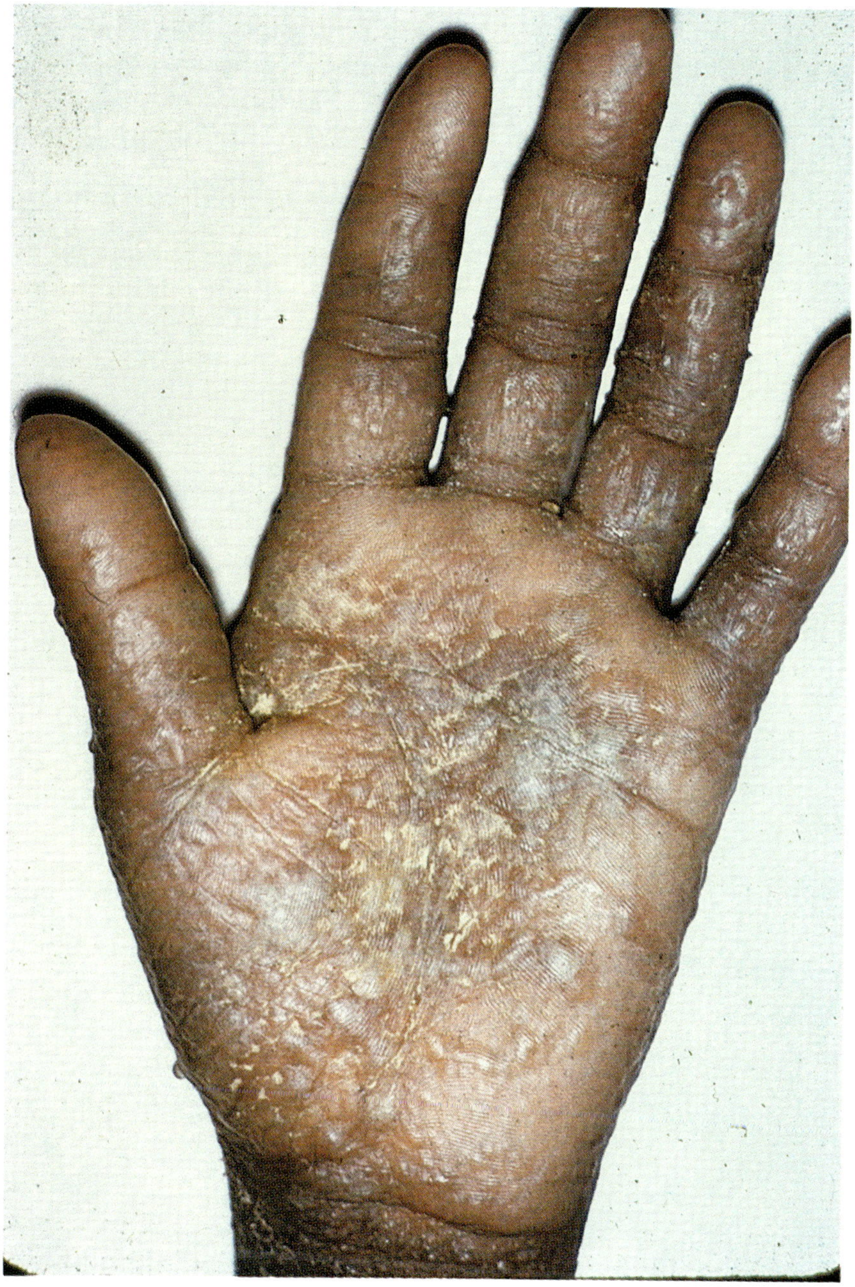

ALKALINE SOLVENT

INSECTICIDE (VAPONA)

HISTORY

A 63-year-old telephone repair person was required to insert an insecticide (DDVP, trade name Vapona, made by Ciba-Geigy Ltd.) into holes drilled into telephone poles. He did not wear gloves. By that evening he noticed burning and itching of the skin, and later fissuring and scaling. Patch testing to standard and vehicle-preservative allergens was negative.

RESOLUTION

He remained off work and under treatment with topical corticosteroids for 3 weeks, during which time the skin gradually returned to normal.

CLINICAL COMMENTS

Many instances of contact dermatitis in the workplace result from workers who perform certain jobs without adequate protection. Usually they are provided insufficient or no protective clothing and instruction, but often the workers themselves ignore warnings. DDVP, 2,2-dichloroethenyl dimethyl phosphate, also known as dichlorvos, is a potent fungicide and insecticide. As is true with many other fungicides and insecticides, it is insoluble in water and must be mixed with a solvent such as dichloro methane, 2-propanol, or toluene.

Reference

Hogan DJ: Pesticides and other agricultural chemicals. In Adams RM (ed): Occupational Skin Disease, 2nd ed. Philadelphia, WB Saunders, 1990, pp 542–578.

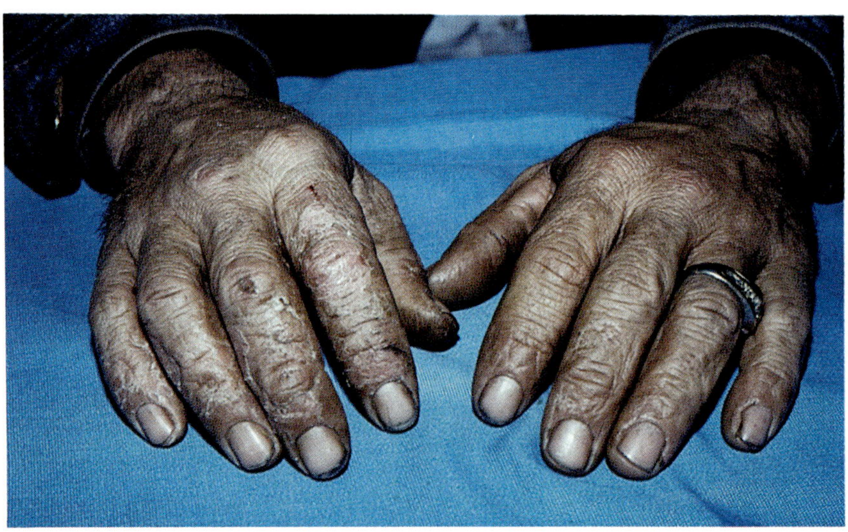

INSECTICIDE

LIGHTER FLUID

HISTORY

A construction worker repairing a bridge in the South Pacific carried a cigarette lighter in his jacket pocket. It leaked lighter fluid one hot afternoon while he was sleeping on a bed. Within hours a blister had formed which required several weeks to heal. Patch testing was not done.

RESOLUTION

This case was referred for consideration of a worker compensation claim. The man was on duty at the time, working under contract for a construction company. Although disputed by his employer, the insurance company agreed to pay for treatment and his time lost from work.

CLINICAL COMMENTS

This case illustrates how extensive and severe blistering can be when there is prolonged skin contact with solvents.

Reference

Shmunes E: Solvents and plasticizers. In Adams RM (ed): Occupational Skin Disease, 2nd ed. Philadelphia, WB Saunders, 1990, pp 439–462.

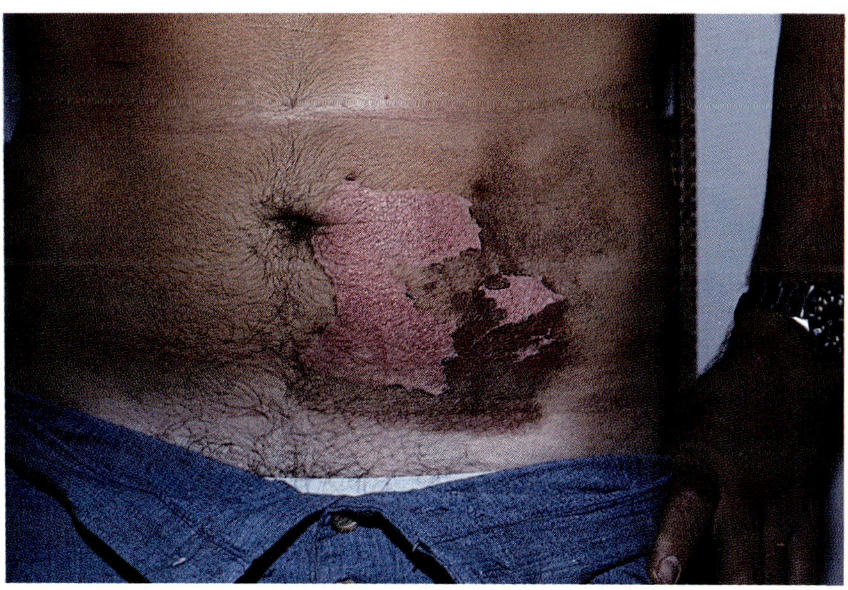

LIGHTER FLUID

ETHYLENE OXIDE

HISTORY

A 63-year-old woman underwent gallbladder surgery at a local hospital. While in the recovery room, extensive areas of redness were noted on her buttocks, back, and legs. Within a few hours blistering and oozing were seen. Initial diagnosis was a localized form of Lyell disease (toxic epidermal necrolysis). On investigation, it was determined that the cause was residue of ethylene oxide used for sterilization of the surgical sheets.

RESOLUTION

The safe level for ethylene oxide gas recommended by the Health Industries Association (HIA) is 200 ppm. Incompletely aerated gowns and sheets should be immediately removed from the sterilizer and washed several times thoroughly with water.

CLINICAL COMMENTS

Ethylene oxide gas is used in many hospitals to clean certain medical devices that cannot be placed in sterilizing solutions or steam autoclaves. Surgical sheets, gowns, and drapes are commonly sterilized by this method. If the machine is not completely aerated following sterilization, residues of highly irritating ethylene oxide may remain.

References

Biro L, Fisher AA, Price E: Ethylene oxide burns, a hospital outbreak involving 19 women. Arch Dermatol 110:924, 1974.

Fisher AA: Ethylene oxide (EO) burns. In Adams RM (ed): Occupational Skin Disease, 2nd ed. Philadelphia, WB Saunders, 1990, pp 17–18.

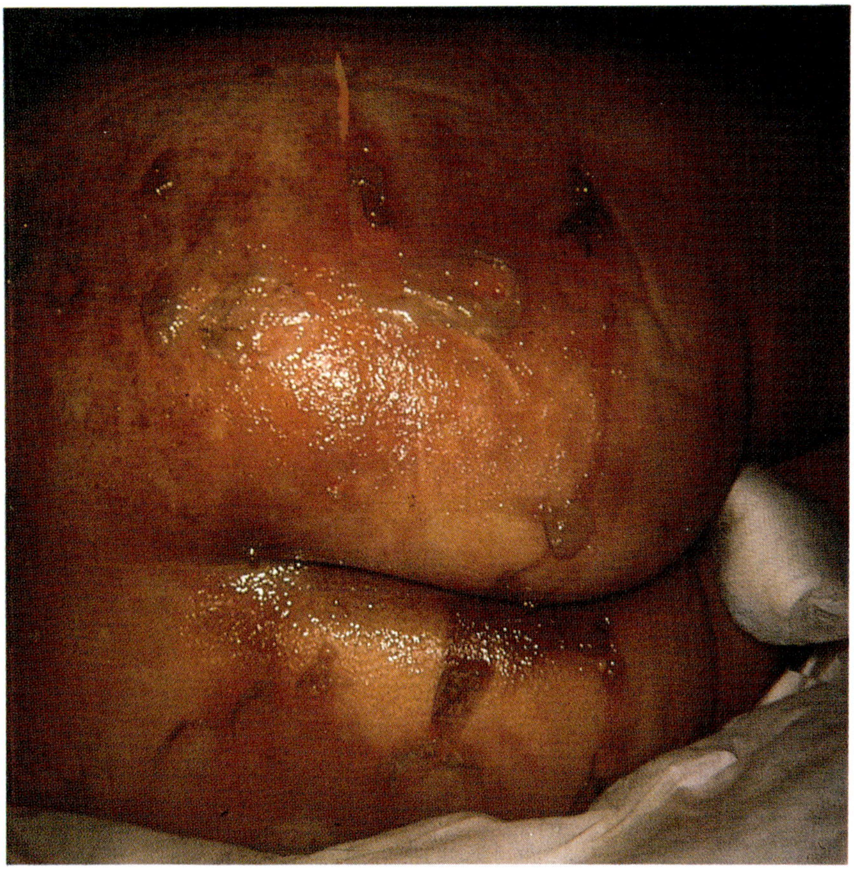

Courtesy of Alexander A. Fisher, M.D.

ETHYLENE OXIDE

HYDROFLUORIC ACID

HISTORY

A young lawyer had purchased a small dry cleaning establishment as an investment. When one of the workers failed to report to work, the lawyer took over his job for a couple of days. Using an "erusticator" he cleaned rust stains from a pair of jeans. He noted slight burning shortly afterwards but 6 hours later experienced severe burning around and under his fingernails. When he was seen, swelling and erythema were present around the fingernails. The pain was severe.

RESOLUTION

Examination of the bottle containing the "erusticator" revealed it consisted of 10% hydrofluoric acid. Treatment by injections, using a 30-gauge needle, of very small amounts of calcium gluconate in and around the fingernails resulted in prompt reduction in pain and resolution of the condition. Destruction of the underlying bone did not occur.

CLINICAL COMMENTS

Hydrofluoric acid produces little evidence of burning on the surface of the skin mainly because of its limited dissociation constant. However, this property permits it to penetrate intact skin, where dissociation into free fluoride and free hydrogen ion takes place in deeper tissues. The fluoride ion is extremely toxic to tissues, with an affinity for bone. Treatment must be prompt following exposure, consisting in injection of 10% calcium gluconate.

Reference

Vance MV: Hydrofluoric acid (HF) burns. In Adams RM (ed): Occupational Skin Disease, 2nd ed. Philadelphia, WB Saunders, 1990, pp 18–21.

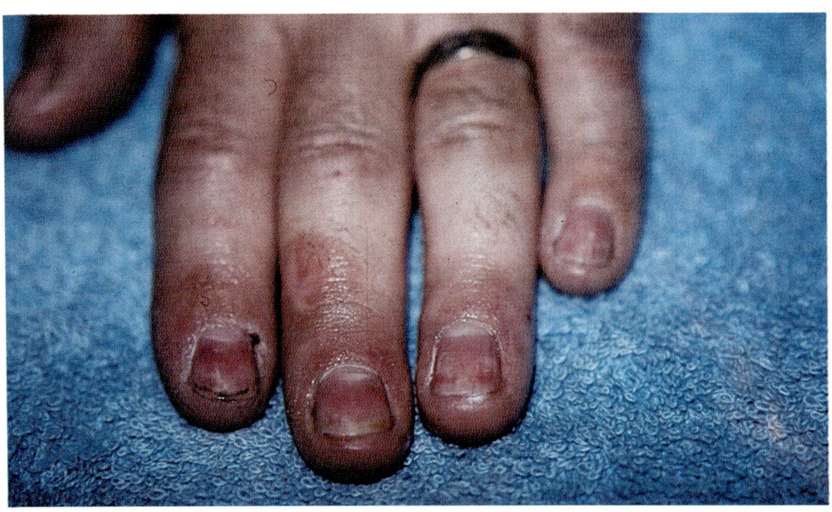

HYDROFLUORIC ACID

TOPICAL MEDICATIONS

HISTORY

For 3 years this 63-year-old woman had applied a large number of topical medications to her lips for "dryness and cracking." Although she was greatly embarrassed by her appearance, she continued searching for new medications and persisted in applying several of her old ones. Initially the dermatitis was thought to be due to either toothpaste or lipstick. When patch testing to a large number of contactants was negative, she was urged to discontinue all topical medication and over-the-counter preparations.

RESOLUTION

After many months of trial and error, she finally discontinued all treatment except a small amount of Vaseline to her lips several times a day. Oral erythromycin was given, and maintenance at BID dosage, combined with strict avoidance of rubbing, slowly cleared the condition. It has now been 1 year since treatment began, and her lip area is completely clear.

CLINICAL COMMENTS

Diagnosis in this case was relatively easy but could only be accomplished after patch testing to rule out contact allergy. The difficulty was encountered in persuading the patient to give up her numerous topical medications and realize the cause of her condition.

Reference

Lyell A: Cutaneous artifactual disease. J Am Acad Dermatol 1:391, 1979.

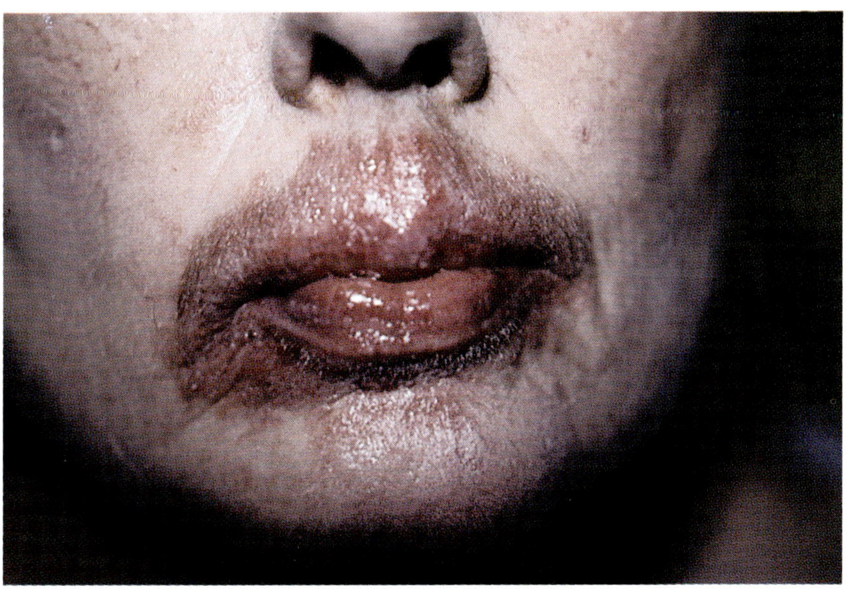

TOPICAL MEDICATIONS

Section XIX

Allergic Contact Dermatitis

COREACTION, NEOSPORIN AND POLYMYXIN B

HISTORY

One week following application of a cream containing polymyxin B to a small area of poison oak dermatitis, an explosive dermatitis developed in this patient, limited mostly to the neck but also appearing on the fingers and face. Patch testing to polymyxin B 3% in petrolatum was strongly positive (*A*).

RESOLUTION

The dermatitis rapidly cleared with appropriate treatment. The patient was cautioned to avoid not only products containing polymyxin B but also bacitracin because of possible cross reaction.

CLINICAL COMMENTS

Both polymyxin B and bacitracin are derived from *Bacillus subtilis,* and both cross react in patients sensitized to one or the other. Neomycin, however, does not cross react with polymyxin B or bacitracin but may "coreact" because of the great frequency in its use, as shown (*B*).

References

Fisher AA: Contact Dermatitis, 3rd ed. Philadelphia, Lea & Febiger, 1986, p 201.
Grandinetti PJ, Fowler JF: Simultaneous contact allergy to neomycin, bacitracin, and polymyxin. J Am Acad Dermatol 23:646, 1990.
van Ketel WG: Polymixin B-sulfate and bacitracin. Contact Dermatitis Newsletter 15:445, 1974.

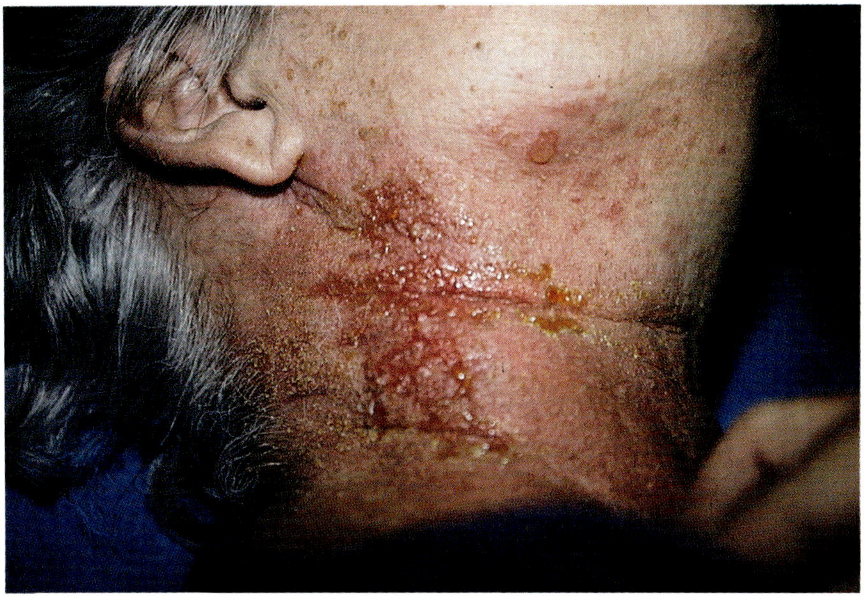

A

NEOSPORIN AND POLYMYXIN B CO-REACTION

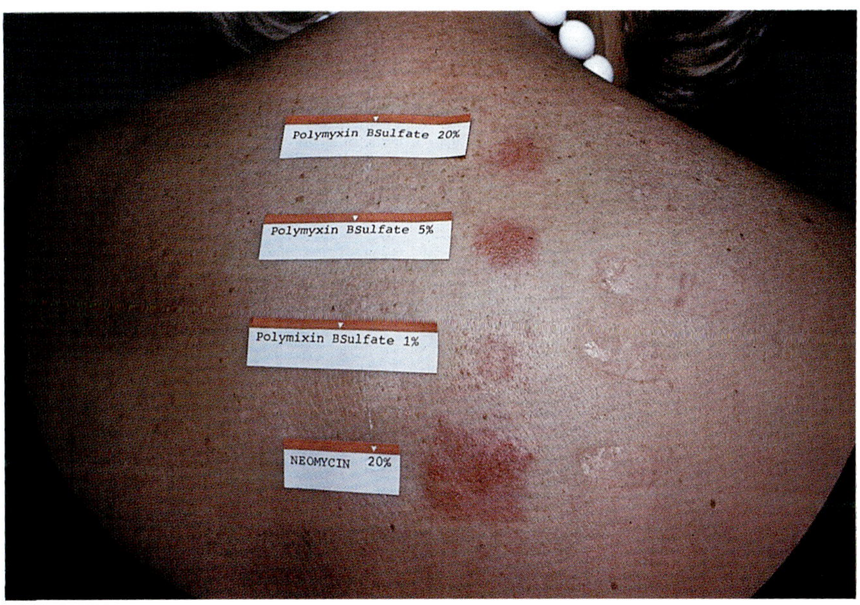

B

NEOMYCIN AND POLYMYXIN B "CO-REACTION"

APPENDIX

ALLERGENS

Allergens are available from
TROLABS
PO Box 1228
D-2057 Reinbek/Hamburg
Germany

The standard North American Patch Test Series is available from:

HERMAL Pharmaceutical Labs, Inc.
Route 145
Oak Hill, New York 12460
(518) 239-6485/(800) HERMAL 1

	Substance	Concentration

European Standard

	Substance	Concentration
1	Potassium Dichromate*	0.5 %
2	Neomycin Sulphate	20 %
3	Thiuram Mix (Tetramethylthiuram Disulphide, Tetraethylthiuram Disulphide, Tetramethylthiuram Monosulphide, Dipentamethylenethiuram Disulphide; 0.25 % each)	1 %
4	Paraphenylenediamine free base	1 %
5	Cobalt Chloride ($CoCl_2$, 6 H_2O)	1 %
6	Benzocaine	5 %
7	Formaldehyde (in water)	1 %
8	Colophony	20 %
9	Quinoline Mix (Clioquinol, Chlorquinaldol; 3 % each)	6 %
10	Balsam of Peru	25 %
11	PPD-Black Rubber Mix** (N-Isopropyl-N'-phenyl Paraphenylenediamine, N-Cyclohexyl-N'-phenyl Paraphenylenediamine, N,N'-Diphenyl Paraphenylenediamine; 0.1 %, 0.25 %, 0.25 %)	0.6 %
12	Wool Alcohols	30 %
13	Mercapto Mix (Mercaptobenzothiazole, N-Cyclohexylbenzothiazyl Sulphenamide, Dibenzothiazyl Disulphide, Morpholinylmercaptobenzothiazole; 0.5 % each)	2 %
14	Epoxy Resin	1 %
15	Paraben Mix (Methyl Parahydroxybenzoate, Ethyl Parahydroxybenzoate, Propyl Parahydroxybenzoate, Butyl Parahydroxybenzoate, Benzyl Parahydroxybenzoate; 3 % each)	15 %
16	Paratertiarybutyl Phenol Formaldehyde Resin (BPF-Resin)	1 %
17	Fragrance Mix ◆ (Cinnamyl Alcohol, Cinnamaldehyde, Eugenol, alpha-Amyl-Cinnamaldehyde, Hydroxycitronellal, Geraniol, Isoeugenol, Oak Moss Absolute; 1 % each)	8 %
18	Ethylenediamine Dihydrochloride	1 %
19	Quaternium 15 (cis-1-(3-Chloroallyl)-3,5,7-triaza-1-azoniaadamantane Chloride)	1 %
20	Nickel Sulphate ($NiSO_4$, 6 H_2O)	5 %
21	5-Chloro-2-methyl-4-isothiazolin-3-one + 2-Methyl-4-isothiazolin-3-one (3:1 in water)	0.01 %
22	Mercaptobenzothiazole (MBT)	2 %
23	Primin***	0.01 %
	complete EUROPEAN STANDARD SET (23 substances) in service and storage box	
	complete EUROPEAN STANDARD SET (23 substances) refill-package	

* slightly irritant; when relevance is in doubt, retest at 0.25 %
** antioxidants in rubber, not related to hair dyes
*** important in only some countries
◆ contains the emulsifier Sorbitan Sesquioleate (E 1703)

The above test sequence has been chosen to make sure that substances that frequently cause cross or concomitant sensitization are not adjacent if the substances are applied vertically in columns of 5.

(Reproduced with permission from Kurt Herrmann, Hermal/Trolabs: Product catalogue. Reinbek/Hamburg, Germany.)

	Substance	Concentration

Antimicrobials, Preservatives

	Substance	Concentration
1	Chlorocresol (PCMC)	1 %
2	Chloroxylenol (PCMX)	1 %
3	Bronopol	0.5 %
4	Imidazolidinyl Urea (Germall 115)	2 %
5	Butyl Hydroxytoluene (BHT)	2 %
6	Butyl Hydroxyanisole (BHA)	2 %
7	Phenylmercuric Acetate (in water)	0.01 %
8	Sorbic Acid	2 %
9	Chlorhexidine Digluconate (in water)	0.5 %
10	Chloramine T (in water)	0.5 %
11	Chloracetamide	0.2 %
12	Glutardialdehyde	1 %
13	1,3,5-Tris(2-hydroxyethyl)-hexahydrotriazine	1 %
14	2-Chloro-N-hydroxy Methylacetamide	0.2 %
15	Thiomersal	0.1 %
16	Phenylmercuric Nitrate (in water)	0.01 %
17	Clioquinol (Chinoform)	5 %
18	Chlorquinaldol	5 %
19	Methyl Parahydroxybenzoate	3 %
20	Ethyl Parahydroxybenzoate	3 %
21	Propyl Parahydroxybenzoate	3 %
22	Butyl Parahydroxybenzoate	3 %
23	Benzyl Parahydroxybenzoate	3 %
24	Benzalkonium Chloride (in water)	0.1 %
25	Hexyl Resorcinol	0.25 %
26	Triclosan	2 %
27	Benzotriazole	1 %

Dental Materials

	Substance	Concentration
1	Benzoyl Peroxide	1 %
2	Tetracaine (Amethocaine) Hydrochloride	1 %
3	Mercury	1 %
4	Copper Sulphate (in water)	1 %
5	Potassium Dicyanoaurate (in water)	0.002 %
6	Methyl Methacrylate	2 %
7	Hydroquinone	1 %
8	Bisphenol A	1 %
9	N,N-Dimethyl-p-Toluidine	2 %
10	Eugenol ◆	1 %
11	Ethyleneglycol Dimethacrylate (EGDMA)	2 %
12	Triethyleneglycol Dimethacrylate (TEGDMA)	2 %
13	BIS-GMA	2 %

Hairdressing

	Substance	Concentration
1	o-Nitro-p-phenylenediamine	1 %
2	Resorcinol	2 %
3	p-Toluenediamine Sulphate	1 %
4	Glyceryl Monothioglycolate	1 %
5	Ammonium Thioglycolate	2.5 %
6	Ammonium Persulphate	2.5 %
7	p-Aminodiphenylamine Hydrochloride	0.25 %
8	Pyrogallol	1 %

Local Anaesthetics

	Substance	Concentration
1	Procaine Hydrochloride	1 %
2	Cinchocaine Hydrochloride (Cincaine)	5 %
3	Tetracaine (Amethocaine) Hydrochloride	1 %
4	Lidocaine Hydrochloride	15 %

	Substance	Concentration

Medicaments

1	Benzoyl Peroxide	1 %
2	Resorcinol	2 %
3	Monobenzone (Hydroquinone Monobenzylether)	1 %
4	Propolis	10 %
5	Tylosin Tartrate	5 %
6	Phenyl Salicylate	1 %
7	Halquinol	1 %
8	Thiamine Hydrochloride (Vit. B_1)	10 %
9	Pyridoxine Hydrochloride (Vit. B_6)	10 %
10	Clioquinol (Chinoform)	5 %
11	Chlorquinaldol	5 %
12	Piperazine	1 %
13	Arnica Tincture ◆	20 %
14	Bacitracin	20 %
15	Chloramphenicol	5 %
16	Gentamycin Sulphate	20 %
17	Nitrofurazone	1 %
18	Propantheline Bromide	5 %
19	Quinine Sulphate	1 %
20	Quinoline Yellow	0.1 %
21	Sulfanilamide	5 %

Metal Compounds

1	Ammoniated Mercury	1 %
2	Mercury	1 %
3	Copper Sulphate (in water)	1 %
4	Potassium Dicyanoaurate (in water)	0.002 %
5	Sodium Thiosulfatoaurate	0.5 %
6	Ammonium Tetrachloroplatinate	0.25 %
7	Palladium Chloride	1 %

Miscellaneous

1	Phosphorus Sesquisulphide	1 %
2	Dioxane	1 %

	Substance	Concentration

Organic Dyes

1	Disperse Orange 3	1 %
2	Disperse Yellow 3	1 %
3	Disperse Red 1	1 %
4	Disperse Red 17	1 %
5	Disperse Blue 3	1 %
6	Eosine	50 %
7	p-Aminophenol	2 %

Perfumes, Flavours

1	Benzyl Salicylate	1 %
2	Clove Oil	2 %
3	Orange Oil	2 %
4	Vanillin	10 %
5	Cinnamyl Alcohol ◆	1 %
6	Cinnamaldehyde ◆	1 %
7	Eugenol ◆	1 %
8	alpha-Amyl-Cinnamaldehyde ◆	1 %
9	Hydroxycitronellal ◆	1 %
10	Geraniol ◆	1 %
11	Isoeugenol ◆	1 %
12	Oak Moss Absolute ◆	1 %
13	Benzaldehyde	5 %
14	Benzylcinnamate	5 %
15	Cedarwood Oil	10 %
16	Eucalyptus Oil	2 %
17	Laurel Oil	2 %
18	Lemon Grass Oil	2 %
19	Lemon Oil	2 %
20	Neroli Oil	2 %
21	Peppermint Oil	2 %
22	Salicylaldehyde	2 %

Substance	Concen-tration

Pesticides

1	Captan	0.1 %
2	Zineb	1 %
3	Captafol (Difolatan®)	0.1 %
4	Maneb	1 %
5	Folpet (Phaltan®)	0.1 %
6	Pyrethrum	2 %
7	Benomyl® (Benlate)	0.1 %
8	Ziram®	1 %

Photoallergens

1	Tribromsalan	1 %
2	6-Methylcoumarin	1 %
3	Chlorpromazine Hydrochloride	0.1 %
4	Fenticlor	1 %
5	Musk Ambrette	5 %
6	Promethazine Hydrochloride	1 %
7	p-Aminobenzoic Acid (PABA)	5 %
8	Bithionol	1 %
9	Hexachlorophene	1 %
10	Tetrachloro Salicylanilide	0.1 %
11	Diphenhydramine Hydrochloride	1 %
12	Musk Ketone	5 %
13	Musk Xylene	5 %
14	Thiourea	0.1 %
15	Triclocarban	1 %

Substance	Concen-tration

Photographic Chemicals

1	Ammonium Persulphate	2.5 %
2	p-Methylaminophenol Sulphate (Metol)	1 %
3	Color Developer CD 2	1 %
4	Color Developer CD 3	1 %
5	Color Developer CD 1	1 %
6	Color Developer CD 4	1 %
7	Color Developer CD 32	1 %
8	Color Developer CD 60	1 %
9	1-Phenyl-3-pyrazolidinone (Phenidone)	1 %
10	Pyrogallol	1 %
11	p-Aminophenol	2 %
12	Hydroquinone	1 %
13	Hydrazine Sulphate	1 %
14	Pyrocatechol	2 %
15	Triphenyl Phosphate	5 %

Plants, Woods

1	alpha-Pinene	15 %
2	Dipentene (dl-Limonene)	2 %
3	Alantolactone (Helenin)	0.1 %
4	Usnic Acid	0.1 %
5	Atranorin	0.5 %
6	Arnica Tincture ◆	20 %

	Substance	Concentration

Plastics, Glues

1	Phenol Formaldehyde Resin, Novolac	5 %
2	Triethylenetetramine	0.5 %
3	4,4'-Diaminodiphenyl Methane	0.5 %
4	Toluenesulphonamide Formaldehyde Resin	10 %
5	Urea Formaldehyde Resin	10 %
6	Melamine Formaldehyde Resin	10 %
7	Phenol Formaldehyde Resin, Resol	5 %
8	Resorcinol Monobenzoate	1 %
9	Diethylenetriamine	0.5 %
10	Isophoronediamine	0.5 %
11	Abitol	10 %
12	alpha-Pinene	15 %
13	Cresylglycidylether	0.25 %
14	Paratertiary Butylcatechol	1 %
15	Paratertiary Butylphenol	2 %
16	Benzoyl Peroxide	1 %
17	Turpentine Oil	10 %
18	Di-n-Butylphthalate	5 %
19	Tricresyl Phosphate	5 %
20	n-Butylglycidylether	0.25 %
21	Phenylglycidylether	0.25 %
22	Diethylphthalate	5 %
23	Diisodecylphthalate	5 %
24	Dimethylphthalate	5 %
25	Diphenylmethane 4,4-Diisocyanate	0.1 %
26	Phenylisocyanate	0.1 %
27	Toluenediisocyanate	0.1 %
28	Triphenylmethane Triisocyanate	0.1 %
29	Triphenyl Phosphate	5 %
30	Di-2-Ethylhexyl-Phthalate	5 %
31	Butyl Acrylate	0.1 %
32	Epichlorohydrin	0.1 %
33	N,N-Dimethyl-p-Toluidine	2 %
34	Abietic Acid	5 %
35	Bisphenol A	1 %

	Substance	Concentration

Rubber Chemicals

1	Monobenzone (Hydroquinone Monobenzylether)	1 %
2	4,4'-Dihydroxybiphenyl	0.1 %
3	Hexamethylenetetramine	2 %
4	Dibenzothiazyl Disulphide	1 %
5	Diphenylthiourea	1 %
6	Ethylenethiourea	1 %
7	Dithiodimorpholine	1 %
8	Dibutylthiourea	1 %
9	Diethylthiourea	1 %
10	N-Cyclohexylbenzothiazyl Sulphenamide (CBS)	1 %
11	1,3-Diphenylguanidine (DPG)	1 %
12	N-Isopropyl-N'-phenyl Paraphenylenediamine (IPPD)	0.1 %
13	Tetramethylthiuram Monosulphide (TMTM)	0.25 %
14	Bis(diethyldithiocarbamato) Zinc (ZDC)	1 %
15	Tetramethylthiuram Disulphide (TMTD)	0.25 %
16	N-Cyclohexyl-N'-phenyl Paraphenylenediamine	0.25 %
17	N,N'-Diphenyl Paraphenylenediamine	0.25 %
18	Morpholinylmercaptobenzothiazole	0.5 %
19	Tetraethylthiuram Disulphide	0.25 %
20	Dipentamethylenethiuram Disulphide	0.25 %
21	Bis(dibutyldithiocarbamato) Zinc	1 %
22	Piperazine	1 %
23	Cyclohexyl Thiophthalimide	1 %

Sunscreen Agents

1	1-(4-Isopropylphenyl)-3-Phenyl-1,3-Propanedione (Eusolex® 8020)	2 %
2	4-tert-Butyl-4'-Methoxy-Dibenzoylmethane (Parsol® 1789)	2 %
3	p-Aminobenzoic Acid	2 %
4	2-Ethylhexyl-p-Dimethylaminobenzoate (Escalol® 507)	2 %
5	2-Ethylhexyl-p-Methoxycinnamate (Parsol® MCX)	2 %
6	3-(4-Methylbenzylidene)-Camphor (Eusolex® 6300)	2 %
7	Oxybenzone (Eusolex® 4360)	2 %
8	Isoamyl p-methoxycinnamate	2 %
9	Benzophenone 4	2 %

Substance	Concentration

Tars, Balsams

1	Pix Lithanthracis (Coal Tar)	3 %
2	Pix Betulae (Birch Tar)	3 %
3	Pix Fagi (Beech Tar)	3 %
4	Pix Oxycedri (Juniper Tar)	3 %
5	Pix Liquida (Pine Tar)	3 %
6	Storax	2 %
7	Balsam of Pine	20 %
8	Balsam of Spruce	20 %
9	Balsam of Tolu	20 %
10	Venice Turpentine	20 %

Textile Finishes

1	Urea Formaldehyde Resin	10 %
2	Melamine Formaldehyde Resin	10 %

Vehicles, Emulsifiers

1	Eucerin®	100 %
2	Trolamine (Triethanolamine)	2.5 %
3	Propyleneglycol	2 %
4	Sorbitan Sesquioleate	20 %
5	Cetylstearylalcohol	20 %
6	Amerchol® L 101	50 %
7	Polyoxyethylene Sorbitan Monopalmitate	10 %
8	Polyoxyethylene Sorbitan Monooleate	10 %

Substance	Concentration

Control

1	White Petrolatum	100 %

Service Items

1	Empty service and storage box for complete EUROPEAN STANDARD SET
2	TROLAB Order Form
3	TROLAB Patient's Test Sheet
4	TROLAB Brochure
5	Handbook: TROLAB Guide to Patch Testing
6	Patch Testing – Points to be observed
7	Questionnaire when a contact allergy is suspected
8	Advice to Patients with Allergic Contact Dermatitis
9	Info sheets for European Standard (23 pads with 25 papers each)
10	Folder test series "Cosmetic Ingredients"

Index

Note: Page numbers in *italics* indicate illustrations; those followed by (t) refer to pages.

E

F

G

H

I

Q

R

S